Neuroanatomy

AN ILLUSTRATED COLOUR TEXT

For Elsevier Churchill Livingstone

Commissioning Editor: Timothy Horne
Senior Development Editor: Ailsa Laing
Project Manager: Jess Thompson
Designer: Kirsteen Wright
Illustration Manager: Bruce Hogarth

Neuroanatomy

FOURTH EDITION

AN ILLUSTRATED COLOUR TEXT

Alan R Crossman PhD DSc
Professor of Anatomy
Faculty of Life Sciences
The University of Manchester
Manchester, UK

David Neary MD FRCP
Professor of Neurology
The University of Manchester
Manchester, UK

Illustrated by Ben Crossman

CHURCHILL LIVINGSTONE

ELSEVIER

EDINBURGH   LONDON   NEW YORK   OXFORD   PHILADELPHIA   ST LOUIS   SYDNEY   TORONTO   2010

CHURCHILL
LIVINGSTONE
ELSEVIER

An imprint of Elsevier Limited

ISBN 978-0-7020-3086-4
  Reprinted 2011

British Library Cataloguing in Publication Data
A catalogue record for this book is available from the British Library

Library of Congress Cataloging in Publication Data
A catalog record for this book is available from the Library of Congress

ELSEVIER your source for books,
journals and multimedia
in the health sciences
www.elsevierhealth.com

Working together to grow
libraries in developing countries

www.elsevier.com | www.bookaid.org | www.sabre.org

ELSEVIER BOOK AID
International Sabre Foundation

The
publisher's
policy is to use
**paper manufactured
from sustainable forests**

Printed in China

Preface to the Fourth Edition

Neuroanatomy is the fundamental cornerstone for understanding nervous system function and dysfunction. In our experience, it is also the area of anatomy that students find both most interesting and most difficult to grasp. It is ironic, therefore, that in many medical schools, the time in the undergraduate curriculum devoted to anatomy, including neuroanatomy, continues to be eroded. There is, thus, an obvious need for a succinct, clear and well-illustrated account of the anatomy of the human nervous system, for medical students. This has been our goal with the new edition of *Neuroanatomy*.

In revising the text, our aims have been to ensure relevance of material and clarity of presentation. To these ends, the degree of detail of neuroanatomical information presented is that which, in our judgement, is necessary to understand how the nervous system works and to provide the basis for the diagnosis and treatment of neurological disorders. As in previous editions, the revised first chapter provides an overview of the entire topic including basic neuroanatomical principles, the main sensory, motor and cognitive systems and the fundamentals of clinical diagnosis of neurological disease.

Anatomy is a highly visual subject and lends itself naturally to the use of high-quality photographs and illustrations to explain both topographical features and internal organisation. We therefore regard the illustrations as particularly important and these have been comprehensively revised and improved for this edition. This considerable task has been undertaken with great skill, insight and enthusiasm by Ben Crossman. Many of the illustrations have been prepared entirely new for this edition and have been introduced to bring further clarity to the text. Many of the photographic images have been skilfully retouched to remove or repair blemishes, or to improve colour and contrast. Working with Ben to transform our elementary sketches, verbal descriptions and, sometimes, ill-formed ideas into the illustrations that enhance this new edition has been a great pleasure and also great fun.

Manchester   **A R Crossman**
2009   **D Neary**

Preface to the First Edition

This book has been written primarily for undergraduate medical students. At the same time, we have borne in mind students following other health science courses where a basic understanding of the nervous system and its major disorders is required, and also students of basic neuroscience, who are invariably intrigued and edified by discussion of the disorders which afflict the human nervous system.

The book has been prepared during a period of widespread debate on, and evolution in, the substance and style of medical education. There are several driving forces for change, one being the recognition that unreasonable and unnecessary demands are often being made of students in the sheer volume of information which they are required to assimilate. This has prompted students, educators and health professionals alike to question, across the whole curriculum, the depth of knowledge which is required by the newly-qualified doctor and the means by which it should be achieved. The General Medical Council has recommended the development of a system-based core curriculum and has emphasised the crucial importance of integration between basic science and clinical medicine. These proposals have been welcomed and amplified, with respect to the teaching of neurology, by the Association of British Neurologists.

No area of medical science lends itself better than neuroscience to such a system-based, integrated approach and this has been the principal philosophy guiding the preparation of this book. Neuroscience, with all its sub-specialities both basic and clinical, is an enormous field where the growth of knowledge through research is exponential. This creates a great challenge to the medical educator in selecting what should comprise the core curriculum. It also signifies the potential for future advances in the diagnosis, prevention and treatment of neurological disease, recognised by the designation of the 1990s as the 'Decade of the Brain'.

Neuroanatomy is the cornerstone upon which is built an understanding of the nervous system and its disorders. The aim of this book, therefore, is to provide a clear and concise account of the anatomy of the human nervous system in sufficient detail to understand its main functions and the common disorders by which it is affected. An important feature of the book is the integration of neuroanatomy with illustrative clinical material. This has been done in order to show how a knowledge of neuroanatomy can help in the understanding of clinical symptoms and also to emphasise those areas of neuroanatomy which are particularly relevant to human neurological disease. We have introduced clinical concepts in the most elementary way to give a broad outline of the aetiology of nervous disease and the link with clinical diagnostic methods. Clinical material has been integrated as closely as possible with the relevant neuroanatomy. Furthermore, the clinical text has been boxed so that it is readily identifiable and can be easily selected to review or pass over. Each chapter also contains boxed summaries. The purpose of these is to assist the reader in identifying key points and as an aid to revision.

Both neuroanatomy and clinical medicine are new to the student first entering medical school. By studying the introductory chapter and the summaries of later, more detailed, chapters the student will gain an overview of the scope and extent of the subject of neuroanatomy and will be introduced to the basic concepts underlying the clinical diagnosis of neurological disease. For those unfamiliar with clinical terminology a glossary has been provided to explain the meaning of commonly used expressions. As more detailed knowledge of neuroanatomy is gained, this will be enhanced and illuminated by reference to the selected clinical material which exemplifies the relevance of neuroanatomy to clinical neurology. Later, when students enter neurological training, they need to refresh in their minds the basic principles of neuroanatomy and link these to clinical diagnostic methods. At this time, the systematic study of patients with individual neurological diseases can be greatly enhanced by returning to the detailed anatomy of diseased structures.

Manchester	**A R Crossman**
1995	**D Neary**

Acknowledgements

We are indebted to Professor David J Brooks, Dr Marco Catani, Professor Paul D Griffiths, Professor Alan Jackson, Professor David Mann, Dr R Anne McKinney and Dr Gary C Schoenwolf for providing scans and other images. We are also most grateful to Dr Adrianne Noe and Archibald J Fobbs for providing images of brain sections from the Yakovlev-Haleem Collection and to Timothy Jones, MR Product Specialist, for providing MR scans courtesy of GE Healthcare. We would also like to thank academic colleagues and students around the world who have sent constructive comments and suggestions.

The authors greatly appreciate the continued interest of the publishers in *Neuroanatomy* and the support and encouragement from colleagues at Elsevier Limited, particularly Publishing Manager Timothy Horne, Senior Development Editor Ailsa Laing and Illustration Manager Bruce Hogarth, in the preparation of this 4th edition.

Manchester   A R Crossman
2009   D Neary

Contents

Chapter 1
Introduction and overview

The human nervous system is the most complex and versatile achievement of evolution. The nervous system of all animals functions to detect changes in the external and internal environments and to bring about appropriate responses in muscles, organs and glands. With the ascent of the evolutionary scale there is, in addition, an increasing capacity for 'higher functions' of the nervous system, such as learning, memory, cognition and, ultimately, self-awareness, intellect and personality. The anatomical, physiological, biochemical and molecular basis of neural function are areas of intense research activity in both the basic and clinical sciences. While a great deal is known about how the nervous system works, much still awaits elucidation.

The nervous system can be damaged by inherited or developmental abnormalities, by disease processes and by traumatic injury. The prevention, diagnosis and treatment of neurological disorders are, therefore, of immense socioeconomic importance. An understanding of neuroanatomy and its correlation with function and dysfunction remains fundamental to the contemporary practice of clinical neuroscience and to the prospect of future advances in prevention and treatment of neurological disorders.

Components and organisation of the nervous system

Neurones and neuroglia

The basic structural and functional unit of the nervous system is the **nerve cell** or **neurone** (Figs 1.1, 1.2), of which the human nervous system is estimated to contain about 10^{10}. The functions of the neurone are to receive and integrate incoming information from **sensory receptors** or other neurones and to transmit information to other neurones or **effector organs**. Neuronal structure is highly specialised to fulfil these functions. Each neurone is a separate entity with a limiting cell membrane. Information is passed between neurones at specialised regions called **synapses** where the membranes of adjacent cells are in close apposition (Fig. 1.1).

There is wide diversity in the shape and size of neurones in different parts of the nervous system, but all share certain common characteristics. There is a single cell body from which a variable number of branching processes emerge. Most of these processes are receptive in function and are known as **dendrites**. They possess synaptic specialisations, sometimes many thousands of them, through which they receive information from other nerve cells. In sensory neurones, the dendrites may be further specialised to detect changes in the external or internal environment. One of the processes leaving the cell body is called the **axon** (nerve fibre) and this carries information away from the cell body. Axons are highly variable in length and may divide into several branches, or collaterals, through which information can be distributed to a number of different destinations simultaneously. At the end of the axon, synaptic specialisations called nerve terminals (presynaptic endings; **terminal boutons**) occur; from these, information is transferred to the dendrites of other neurones.

Information is coded within neurones by changes in electrical energy. The neurone at rest possesses an electrical potential (the **resting potential**) across its membrane of the order of 60–70 millivolts (mV), the inside being negative with respect to the outside. When a neurone is stimulated or excited above a certain threshold level, there is a brief reversal of the polarity of its membrane potential, termed the **action potential**. Action potentials are propagated down the axon and invade the nerve terminals. Transmission of information between neurones almost always occurs by chemical rather than by electrical means.

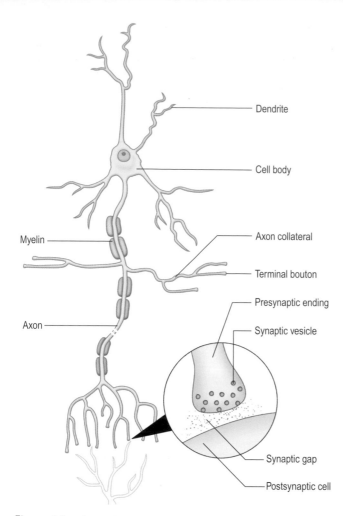

Figure 1.1 **Schematic representation of the basic structure of the neurone and the synapse.**

Figure 1.2 **Pseudocoloured three-dimensional reconstruction of a neurone from the hippocampus, imaged by confocal laser scanning microscopy.** One of the processes at the base of the neurone is the axon. (Courtesy of Dr R A McKinney, Brain Research Institute, University of Zurich, Switzerland.)

Invasion of nerve terminals by an action potential causes the release of specific chemical agents that are stored in **synaptic vesicles** in the presynaptic ending. These chemicals are known as **neurotransmitters** and they diffuse across the narrow gap between pre- and postsynaptic membranes to bind to receptors on the postsynaptic cell, inducing changes in the membrane potential. The change may be either to depolarise the membrane, thus moving towards the threshold for production of action potentials, or to hyperpolarise and, thus, stabilise the cell.

The other major cellular components of the nervous system are **neuroglial cells**, or **glia**, which outnumber neurones by an order of magnitude. Unlike neurones, neuroglia do not have a direct role in information processing but they fulfil a number of ancillary roles essential for the normal functioning of nerve cells. Three main types of neuroglial cell are recognised:

1. **Oligodendroglia** (oligodendrocytes), which form the **myelin sheath** that surrounds many neuronal axons (Fig. 1.1), conferring an increased rate of conduction of action potentials.
2. **Astroglia** (astrocytes), which are thought to form a selectively permeable barrier between the circulatory system and the neurones of the brain and spinal cord. This is known as the 'blood–brain barrier' and has a protective function.

3. **Microglia**, which have a phagocytic role in the local tissue response to nervous system damage.

Central and peripheral nervous systems

The nervous system (Fig. 1.3) is divided into the **central nervous system (CNS)** and the **peripheral nervous system (PNS)**. The central nervous system consists of the **brain** and **spinal cord**, lying within the protection of the cranium and vertebral column, respectively. This is the most complex part of the nervous system. It contains the majority of nerve cell bodies and synaptic connections. The peripheral nervous system constitutes the link between the CNS and structures in the periphery of the body, from which it receives sensory information and to which it sends controlling impulses. The peripheral nervous system consists of nerves joined to the brain and spinal cord (**cranial** and **spinal nerves**) and their ramifications within the body. Spinal nerves serving the upper or lower limbs coalesce to form the **brachial** or **lumbar plexus**, respectively, within which fibres are redistributed into named **peripheral nerves**. The PNS also includes some groups of peripherally located nerve cell bodies that are aggregated within structures called **ganglia**.

Autonomic nervous system

Neurones that detect changes in, and control the activity of, the viscera are collectively referred to as the autonomic nervous system (ANS). Its components are present in both the central and peripheral nervous systems. The autonomic nervous system is divided into two anatomically and functionally distinct parts, namely the **sympathetic** and **parasympathetic** divisions, which generally have opposing (antagonistic) effects on the structures that they innervate. The autonomic nervous system innervates smooth muscle, cardiac muscle and secretory glands. It is an important part of the homeostatic mechanisms that control the internal environment of the body.

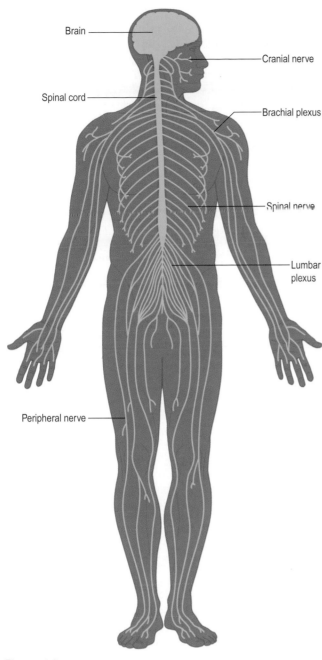

Brain

Cranial nerve

Spinal cord

Brachial plexus

Spinal nerve

Lumbar plexus

Peripheral nerve

Figure 1.3 **Central and peripheral nervous systems.**

Afferent neurones, efferent neurones and interneurones

Nerve cells that carry information from peripheral receptors to the CNS are referred to as **afferent neurones** (Fig. 1.4). If the information that they carry ultimately reaches a conscious level, they are also called **sensory neurones**. **Efferent neurones** carry impulses away from the CNS and if they innervate skeletal muscle to cause movement they are also referred to as **motor neurones**. The vast majority of neurones, however, are located entirely within the CNS and are referred to as **interneurones** (the alternative terms internuncial, or relay, neurones are sometimes used). The terms 'afferent' and 'efferent' are also commonly used to denote the polarity of projections to and from structures within the CNS, even though the projections are entirely contained within the brain and spinal cord. The projections to and from the cerebral cortex, for example, are referred to as cortical afferents and efferents, respectively.

Grey and white matter, nuclei and tracts

The CNS is a highly heterogeneous structure in terms of the distribution of nerve cell bodies and their processes (Fig. 1.5). Some regions are relatively enriched in nerve cell bodies (e.g. the central portion of the spinal cord and the surface of the cerebral hemisphere) and are referred to as **grey matter**. Other regions contain mostly nerve processes (usually axons). These are often myelinated (ensheathed in myelin), which confers a paler coloration – hence the term **white matter**.

Nerve cell bodies with similar anatomical connections and functions (e.g. the motor neurones innervating a group of related muscles) tend to be located together in groups called **nuclei**. Similarly, nerve processes sharing common connections and functions tend to follow the same course, running in **pathways** or **tracts** (Fig. 1.5 and see Fig. 1.19).

Decussation of sensory and motor pathways

It is a general principle of the organisation of the CNS that pathways conveying sensory information to a conscious level (the cerebral hemisphere) cross over, or **decussate**, from one side of the CNS to the other. The same is true of

---

Components and organisation of the nervous system

- The structural and functional unit of the nervous system is the nerve cell, or neurone. Neurones have a resting membrane potential of about −70 mV.
- A neurone receives information primarily through its dendrites and passes this on by action potentials, which are carried away from the cell body by the axon.
- Information is passed between neurones at synapses by release of neurotransmitters from presynaptic terminals; these act upon receptors in the postsynaptic membrane to cause either depolarisation or hyperpolarisation of the postsynaptic cell.
- Neuroglial cells are more numerous than nerve cells but have ancillary roles and are not directly involved in information processing.
- Oligodendrocytes form the myelin sheath that surrounds axons and increases their rate of conduction.
- Astrocytes may form the blood–brain barrier.
- Microglia have a phagocytic function when the nervous system is damaged.
- The nervous system is divided into the central nervous system (CNS), which consists of the brain and spinal cord, and the peripheral nervous system (PNS), which consists of cranial and spinal nerves and their ramifications.
- The autonomic nervous system (ANS) innervates visceral structures and is important in homeostasis of the internal environment.
- Individual neurones may be defined as either afferent or efferent with respect to the CNS, or as interneurones.
- Within the CNS, areas rich in either nerve cell bodies or nerve fibres constitute grey and white matter, respectively.
- Clusters of cell bodies with similar functions are known as nuclei.
- Tracts, or pathways, of nerve fibres link distant regions.
- Generally, ascending sensory and descending motor pathways in the CNS decussate along their course, so that each side of the brain is functionally associated with the contralateral half of the body.

descending pathways from the cerebral hemisphere that control movement. Therefore, in general, each cerebral hemisphere perceives sensations from, and controls the movements of, the opposite (contralateral) side of the body.

Development of the central nervous system

By the beginning of the second week of human embryonic development, three germ cell layers become established: ectoderm, mesoderm and endoderm. Subsequently, these

Afferent nerve ending

Afferent neurone

Interneurone

Efferent neurone

Efferent nerve ending

Figure 1.4 **The general arrangement of afferent, efferent and interneurones.**

each give rise to particular tissues and organs in the adult. The ectoderm gives rise to the skin and the nervous system. The mesoderm forms skeletal, muscular and connective tissues. The endoderm gives rise to the alimentary, respiratory and genitourinary tracts. The process of formation of the embryonic nervous system is referred to as **neurulation**. During the third week of embryonic development, the dorsal midline ectoderm undergoes thickening to form the **neural plate** (Figs 1.6, 1.7). The lateral margins of the neural plate become elevated, forming **neural folds** on either side of a longitudinal, midline depression, the **neural groove**. The neural folds then become apposed and fuse together, thus sealing the neural groove and creating the **neural tube**. Some cells from the apices of the neural folds become separated to form groups lying dorsolateral to the neural tube. These are known as the **neural crests**. The formation of the neural tube is complete by about the middle of the fourth week of embryonic development.

Enormous growth, distortion and cellular differentiation occur during the subsequent transformation of the neural tube into the adult CNS. This is maximal in the rostral part, which develops into the brain, the caudal portion becoming the spinal cord. The central cavity within the neural tube becomes the central canal of the spinal cord and the ventricles of the brain. The neural crests form the sensory ganglia of spinal and cranial nerves, and also the autonomic ganglia.

As development continues, a longitudinal groove, the **sulcus limitans**, appears on the inner surface of the lateral walls of the embryonic spinal cord and caudal part of the brain (Fig. 1.8A). The dorsal and ventral cell groupings thus delineated are referred to as the **alar plate** and the **basal**

Subcortical nuclei

Ascending and descending tracts

Cerebral hemisphere

Grey matter

White matter

Brain stem

Figure 1.5 **Coronal section through the brain illustrating the distribution of grey and white matter.** The section has been stained by Mulligan's technique, which colours grey matter blue, leaving white matter relatively unstained.

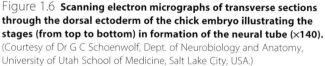

Figure 1.6 **Scanning electron micrographs of transverse sections through the dorsal ectoderm of the chick embryo illustrating the stages (from top to bottom) in formation of the neural tube (×140).** (Courtesy of Dr G C Schoenwolf, Dept. of Neurobiology and Anatomy, University of Utah School of Medicine, Salt Lake City, USA.)

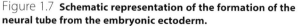

Figure 1.7 **Schematic representation of the formation of the neural tube from the embryonic ectoderm.**

plate, respectively. Nerve cells that develop within the alar plate have predominantly sensory functions, while those in the basal plate are predominantly motor. Further development also brings about the differentiation of grey and white matter. The grey matter is located centrally around the central canal, with white matter forming an outer coat. This basic developmental pattern can still easily be recognised in the adult spinal cord (Fig. 1.8B).

During embryonic development, the rostral portion of the neural tube undergoes massive differentiation and growth to form the brain (Fig. 1.9). By about the fifth week, three **primary brain vesicles** can be identified: the **prosencephalon** (forebrain), **mesencephalon** (midbrain)

and **rhombencephalon** (hindbrain). The longitudinal axis of the developing CNS (neuraxis) does not remain straight but is bent by a midbrain or cephalic flexure, occurring at the junction of midbrain and forebrain, and a cervical flexure between the brain and the spinal cord.

By the seventh week, further differentiation distinguishes five **secondary brain vesicles** produced by division of the prosencephalon into the **telencephalon** and **diencephalon** and division of the rhombencephalon into

Figure 1.11 **Photographs of the brain. (A)** Lateral aspect; **(B)** median sagittal section; **(C)** dorsal aspect; **(D)** ventral aspect.

Figure 1.12 **Principal subdivisions and some important landmarks in the mature brain. (A)** Median sagittal section; **(B)** ventral aspect. Cranial nerves are indicated in yellow.

Overview of the anatomy of the central nervous system

Coverings and blood supply

The brain and spinal cord are supported and protected by the bones of the skull and vertebral column, respectively. Within these bony coverings, the CNS is entirely ensheathed by three layers of membranes, called the **meninges** (Fig. 1.13). The outermost membrane is the **dura mater**, a tough, fibrous coat that surrounds the brain and spinal cord like a loose-fitting bag. The spinal dura and much of the cranial dura are separate from the periosteum, which lines the surrounding bones. At certain locations, however, such as the floor of the cranial cavity, the dura and periosteum are fused and the cranial dura is tightly adherent to the interior of the skull. Two large sheets of dura project into the cranial cavity, incompletely dividing it

into compartments (Fig. 1.14). The **falx cerebri** lies in the sagittal plane between the two cerebral hemispheres. Its free border lies above the corpus callosum. The **tentorium cerebelli** is oriented horizontally, lying beneath the occipital lobes of the cerebral hemispheres and above the cerebellum. The dura mater can be regarded as consisting of two layers. These are fused together except in certain locations, where they become separated to form spaces, the **dural venous sinuses**, which serve as channels for the venous drainage of the brain. Important dural sinuses occur:

- on the floor of the cranial cavity
- along the lines of attachment of the falx cerebri and tentorium cerebelli to the interior of the skull (superior sagittal sinus, Fig. 1.14; transverse sinus Figs 7.9, 7.10)
- along the line of attachment of the falx cerebri and tentorium cerebelli to one another (straight sinus Figs 7.9, 7.10).

Skin

Bone

Dura mater

Arachnoid mater

Subarachnoid space

Trabeculae

Pia mater

Blood vessel

Cerebral cortex

White matter

Figure 1.13 **A section through the skull, illustrating the relationships between the meninges and the CNS.**

Falx cerebri

Superior sagittal sinus

Corpus callosum

Tentorium cerebelli
(containing straight sinus)

Cerebellum

Brain stem

Figure 1.14 **Parasagittal section of the head showing the disposition of the falx cerebri and tentorium cerebelli.**

Coverings and blood supply of the central nervous system

- The brain and spinal cord are invested by three meningeal layers: the dura mater, arachnoid mater and pia mater.
- Two sheets of cranial dura mater, the falx cerebri and tentorium cerebelli, incompletely divide the cranial cavity into compartments.
- The cranial dura mater contains dural venous sinuses, which act as channels for the venous drainage of the brain.

- Beneath the arachnoid mater lies the subarachnoid space in which cerebrospinal fluid (CSF) circulates.
- The brain is supplied with blood by the internal carotid and vertebral arteries.
- The spinal cord is supplied by vessels arising from the vertebral arteries, reinforced by radicular arteries derived from segmental vessels.

Beneath the dura lies the **arachnoid mater**, the two being separated by a thin **subdural space**. The arachnoid is a translucent, collagenous membrane that, like the dura, loosely envelops the brain and spinal cord. The innermost of the meninges is the **pia mater**, a delicate membrane of microscopic thickness that is firmly adherent to the surface of the brain and spinal cord, closely following their contours. Between the arachnoid and pia is the **subarachnoid space** through which CSF circulates.

The brain is supplied with arterial blood by the **internal carotid** and **vertebral arteries**, which anastomose to form the **circulus arteriosus** (circle of Willis) on the base of the brain. The spinal cord is supplied by vessels arising from the vertebral arteries, reinforced by **radicular arteries** derived from segmental vessels. The arteries and veins serving the CNS run for part of their course within the subarachnoid space (Fig. 1.13). The meninges are supplied by a number of vessels, the most significant intracranial one being the **middle meningeal artery**, which ramifies extensively between the skull and dura mater overlying the lateral aspect of the cerebral hemisphere.

Anatomy of the spinal cord

The spinal cord lies within the **vertebral** (spinal) **canal** of the vertebral column and is continuous rostrally with the medulla oblongata of the brain stem (Fig. 1.15). The spinal cord receives information from, and controls, the trunk and limbs. This is achieved through 31 pairs of **spinal nerves** that join the cord at intervals along its length and contain afferent and efferent nerve fibres connecting with structures in the periphery. Near to the cord, the spinal nerves divide into **dorsal** and **ventral roots**, which attach to the cord along its dorsolateral and ventrolateral borders, respectively (Fig. 1.16). The dorsal roots carry afferent fibres, the cell bodies of which are located in **dorsal root ganglia**. The ventral roots carry efferent fibres with cell bodies lying within the spinal grey matter. Spinal nerves leave the vertebral canal through small holes, called **intervertebral foramina**, located between adjacent vertebrae. Because of a difference in the rates of growth of the spinal cord and vertebral column during development, the spinal cord in the adult does not extend the full length of the vertebral canal, but ends at the level of the intervertebral disc between L1 and L2. The lumbar and sacral spinal nerves, therefore, descend in a leash-like arrangement, the **cauda equina** (Fig. 1.15), to reach their exit foramina.

The spinal cord is a relatively undifferentiated structure compared with the brain. Consequently, the basic principles of organisation, established early in embryonic development, can be readily identified even in the adult human cord (Fig. 1.16). The spinal cord is approximately cylindrical in shape, containing at its centre a vestigial **central canal**. The separation of cell bodies from nerve fibres gives a characteristic 'H' or 'butterfly' shape to the central core of grey matter that surrounds the central canal. Four extensions of the central grey matter project dorsolaterally and ventrolaterally towards the lines of attachment of the dorsal and ventral roots of the spinal nerves. These are known as **dorsal horns** and **ventral horns**, respectively. The dorsal horn is the site of termination of many afferent neurones, conveying impulses from sensory receptors throughout the body, and is the site of origin of ascending pathways carrying sensory impulses to the brain. The ventral horn contains motor neurones that innervate

Figure 1.15 **Dorsal aspect of the spinal cord *in situ*.**

Labels: Brain stem; Dorsal roots of spinal nerve; Spinal cord; Cauda equina

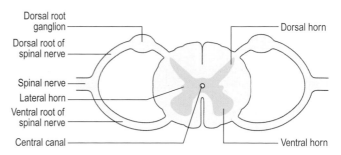

Figure 1.16 **Schematic diagram of a transverse section through the spinal cord, showing the attachment of spinal nerve roots and the arrangement of grey and white matter.**

Labels: Dorsal root ganglion; Dorsal root of spinal nerve; Spinal nerve; Lateral horn; Ventral root of spinal nerve; Central canal; Dorsal horn; Ventral horn

skeletal muscle. In addition, at thoracic and upper lumbar levels of the cord only, another, smaller, collection of cell bodies comprises the **lateral horn**, which contains preganglionic neurones belonging to the sympathetic division of the autonomic nervous system.

Figure 1.17 **Transverse section through the spinal cord showing the locations of the principal ascending (left side) and descending (right side) nerve fibre tracts.**

The periphery of the cord consists of white matter that contains longitudinally running nerve fibres. These are organised into a series of **ascending tracts**, which carry information from the trunk and limbs to the brain, and **descending tracts**, by which the brain controls the activities of neurones in the spinal cord (Fig. 1.17). The principal ascending tracts are the **dorsal columns** (fasciculus gracilis and fasciculus cuneatus), which carry fine touch and proprioception, the **spinothalamic tracts**, which carry pain, temperature, coarse touch and pressure, and the **spinocerebellar tracts**, which carry information from muscle and joint receptors to the cerebellum. Amongst the descending tracts, one of the most important is the **lateral corticospinal tract**, which controls skilled voluntary movements.

Anatomy of the spinal cord

- The spinal cord lies within the vertebral canal. It bears 31 pairs of spinal nerves through which it receives fibres from, and sends fibres to, the periphery.
- Near the cord, spinal nerves divide to form dorsal and ventral roots; dorsal roots carry afferent fibres with cell bodies in dorsal root ganglia, and ventral roots carry efferent fibres.
- The spinal cord consists of a central core of grey matter, containing nerve cell bodies, and an outer layer of white matter or nerve fibres.
- Within the grey matter, the dorsal horn contains sensory neurones, the ventral horn contains motor neurones and the lateral horn contains preganglionic sympathetic neurones.
- Within the white matter run ascending and descending nerve fibre tracts, which link the spinal cord with the brain.
- The principal ascending tracts are the dorsal columns, the spinothalamic tracts and the spinocerebellar tracts. The corticospinal tract is an important descending tract.

Anatomy of the brain
Major features and landmarks
The brain is dominated by the cerebral hemispheres (Figs 1.11, 1.12). These have a highly convoluted outer mantle of grey matter and an inner core of white matter. Certain of the surface convolutions have specific sensory or motor functions, described below. The two cerebral hemispheres are incompletely separated by the **great longitudinal fissure**. The fissure is normally occupied by the falx cerebri and in its depths lies the **corpus callosum**, containing commissural fibres that unite corresponding regions of the two hemispheres.

The brain stem can be seen clearly when the brain is viewed ventrally, although the relationships of the midbrain are best illustrated in sagittal section. The brain stem is the origin of cranial nerves III–XII. Dorsal (posterior) to the brain stem is located the cerebellum. The tentorium cerebelli normally lies between the cerebellum and the posterior part (occipital lobes) of the cerebral hemispheres.

Ventricular system
The highly simplified plan of the basic brain, described above, is a useful one on which to consider the general disposition of the ventricular system (Figs 1.10, 1.12, 1.18). As the central canal of the spinal cord ascends into the brain stem it moves progressively in a dorsal direction, eventually opening out to form a shallow, rhomboid-shaped depression on the dorsal surface of the medulla and pons (the hindbrain portion of the brain stem) beneath the cerebellum. This is the **fourth ventricle**.

At the rostral border of the pons, the walls of the fourth ventricle converge, forming once again a narrow tube, the **cerebral aqueduct**. The cerebral aqueduct dives into the substance of the brain stem running the length of the midbrain beneath the inferior and superior colliculi. At the junction of midbrain and forebrain, the aqueduct opens into the **third ventricle**, a slit-like chamber, narrow from side-to-side but extensive in dorsoventral and rostrocaudal dimensions. The lateral walls of the third ventricle are formed by the thalamus and hypothalamus of the diencephalon. Near the rostral end of the third ventricle a small aperture, the **interventricular foramen** (foramen of Monro), communicates with an extensive chamber, the **lateral ventricle**, within each cerebral hemisphere. The ventricular system contains CSF, which is secreted by the **choroid plexus**.

Brain stem
When the brain is viewed externally, the large cerebral hemispheres obscure many other structures, but a median sagittal section (Figs 1.11B, 1.12A) reveals most of the main features of the basic brain. The brain stem can be clearly seen on both a median sagittal section and a ventral view (Figs 1.11, 1.12) of the brain. The brain stem consists of the medulla oblongata, pons and midbrain.

The brain stem forms only a small proportion of the entire brain but it is crucially important. Through it pass ascending and descending nerve fibre tracts linking the brain and spinal cord (Fig. 1.19). These carry sensory information from, and permit movement of, the trunk and limbs. The brain stem also contains the sites of origin and termination of many of the cranial nerves through which the brain innervates the head. Moreover, within the brain stem lie centres controlling vital functions such as respiration, the cardiovascular system and the level of consciousness.

The medulla oblongata is continuous caudally with the spinal cord and extends rostrally as far as the pons. The latter junction can clearly be seen on ventral or sagittal views since the ventral part of the pons forms a prominent bulge on the surface of the brain stem. In sagittal section (Figs 1.11B, 1.12A), the lumen of the fourth ventricle is apparent between the pons and medulla ventrally and the cerebellum dorsally, into which its tent-shaped roof extends.

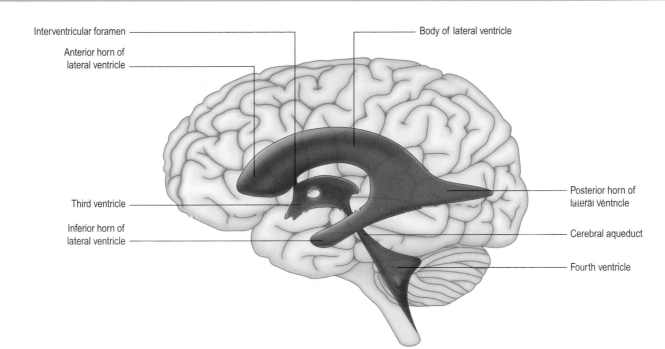

Interventricular foramen

Anterior horn of
lateral ventricle

Body of lateral ventricle

Third ventricle

Inferior horn of
lateral ventricle

Posterior horn of
lateral ventricle

Cerebral aqueduct

Fourth ventricle

Figure 1.18 **The cerebral ventricular system.**

Fourth ventricle

Vestibular nuclei

Hypoglossal nucleus

Inferior cerebellar peduncle

Medial lemniscus

Pyramid

Figure 1.19 **Transverse section through the brain stem at the level of the medulla oblongata.** The section has been stained by the Weigert–Pal method. Areas rich in nerve fibres stain darkly while areas rich in cell bodies are relatively paler. The pyramid contains descending motor fibres which run from the cerebral cortex to the spinal cord. The medial lemniscus consists of ascending axons carrying sensory information from the limbs to higher centres in the brain. The inferior cerebellar peduncle contains spinocerebellar fibres carrying information from joints and muscles to the cerebellum. The vestibular nuclei are the site of termination of the vestibular nerve. The hypoglossal nucleus is the site of origin of hypoglossal nerve fibres.

Cranial nerves

The brain directly receives sensory information from, and controls the activities of, peripheral structures, principally the head and neck. Afferent and efferent nerve fibres run in 12 pairs of cranial nerves, which are identified by individual names and Roman numerals I–XII. Certain of the cranial nerves contain only sensory or only motor nerve fibres but the majority, like spinal nerves, contain a mixture. The first two cranial nerves (I olfactory, II optic) attach directly to the forebrain and the rest attach to the brain stem. Within the brain stem lie a number of cell body groupings, called the **cranial nerve nuclei.** These are the sites of termination of sensory fibres and the origin of the motor fibres (Fig. 1.19) that run in the cranial nerves.

Cerebellum

The cerebellum is attached to the brain stem by a large mass of nerve fibres that lie lateral to the fourth ventricle on either side. The mass is split nominally into three parts: the **inferior, middle** and **superior cerebellar peduncles**.

These carry nerve fibres between the medulla, pons and midbrain, respectively, and the cerebellum.

The cerebellum consists of an outer layer of grey matter, the cerebellar cortex, surrounding a central core of white matter. The cortical surface is highly convoluted to form a regular pattern of narrow, parallel folds or **folia**. The cerebellar white matter consists of nerve fibres running to and from the cerebellar cortex. The white matter has a characteristic branching, tree-like arrangement in section

(Fig. 1.11B), as its ramifications reach towards the surface. The cerebellum is concerned with the coordination of movement and it operates at an entirely unconscious level.

Rostral to the pons is located the relatively small midbrain. On its dorsal surface can be seen the rounded eminences of the superior and inferior colliculi, beneath which runs the cerebral aqueduct (Figs 1.10–1.12).

Diencephalon and cerebral hemispheres

Rostral to the brain stem lies the forebrain, consisting of the diencephalon and cerebral hemispheres. The diencephalon and cerebral hemisphere on each side of the brain are to a large extent physically separate from their counterparts on the other side, although important cross-connections do exist, as described below. The two sides of the diencephalon are separated by the lumen of the third ventricle, whose lateral walls they constitute.

The diencephalon consists of four main divisions in a dorsoventral direction: the **epithalamus**, **thalamus**, **subthalamus** and **hypothalamus**. The epithalamus is small and its most notable component is the pineal gland, which lies in the midline immediately rostral to the superior colliculi of the midbrain (Fig. 1.12A). The thalamus is by far the largest part of the diencephalon and it forms much of the lateral wall of the third ventricle. The thalamus plays an important part in sensory, motor and cognitive functions and it has extensive reciprocal connections with the cerebral cortex. The subthalamus is a small region lying deep to the ventricular wall. It contains the **subthalamic nucleus** which is closely related functionally to the basal ganglia (Ch. 14). The hypothalamus forms the lower part of the walls and floor of the third ventricle. It is a complex and highly important region because of its involvement in the autonomic nervous system (Ch. 4), the limbic system and the neuroendocrine system (Ch. 16). From the ventral aspect of the hypothalamus in the midline arises the **infundibulum** or pituitary stalk, to which is attached the **pituitary gland** (Fig. 1.12).

The cerebral hemisphere is by far the largest part of the brain. Like the cerebellum, it consists of an outer layer, or cortex, of grey matter and an inner mass of white matter (Figs 1.20, 1.21). In addition, partly buried within the subcortical white matter lie several large masses of cell bodies, collectively referred to as the basal ganglia (Figs 1.5, 1.20, 1.21). The two cerebral hemispheres are separated by a deep midline cleft, the great longitudinal fissure (Fig. 1.20), which accommodates the falx cerebri, a sheet of dura mater reflected from the internal surface of the cranium. In the depths of the fissure lies the corpus callosum (Figs 1.12A, 1.20), a large sheet of transversely running nerve fibres (commissural fibres) that link corresponding areas of the two cerebral cortices.

The cerebral cortex is highly convoluted. This has the effect of maximising the cortical surface area, which is about 1 m^2 for each hemisphere. The convolutions are called **gyri** (singular: gyrus) and the furrows between them are **sulci** (singular: sulcus). Some gyri and sulci have a relatively consistent configuration between individuals and they mark the location of important functional areas.

On the lateral surface of the hemisphere, a deep cleft, the **lateral fissure** (Figs 1.20, 1.22), is an important landmark. This, together with certain sulci, forms boundaries that divide the hemisphere into four **lobes** (Fig. 1.22). The lobes bear the names of the bones of the skull beneath which they lie.

The most anterior part of the cerebral hemisphere is called the **frontal lobe**, the most anterior convexity of which is the **frontal pole**. The posterior boundary of the frontal lobe is the **central sulcus**, which can be identified as a single, continuous furrow running over the entire lateral surface of the hemisphere from the great longitudinal fissure to the lateral fissure. Posterior to the central sulcus lies the **parietal lobe**, which is separated from the **temporal lobe** below by the lateral fissure. The tip of the temporal lobe is called the **temporal pole**. The posterior part of the hemisphere is the **occipital lobe**, ending in the **occipital pole**. The boundaries between parietal and temporal lobes and the occipital lobe are indistinct on the lateral surface of the hemisphere, since they do not correspond to any particular sulci; however, on

Great longitudinal fissure

Lateral ventricle

Caudate nucleus

Internal capsule

Putamen

Globus pallidus

Cerebral cortex

White matter

Corpus callosum

Lateral fissure

Thalamus

Hypothalamus

Third ventricle

Figure 1.20 **Coronal section through the cerebral hemisphere.**

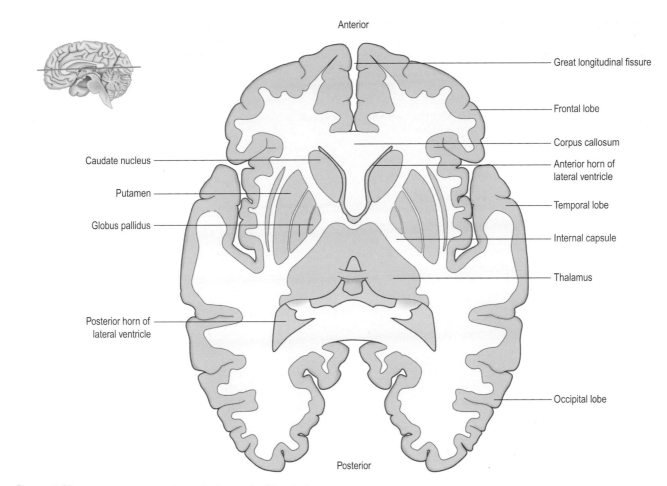

Figure 1.21 **Horizontal section through the cerebral hemisphere.**

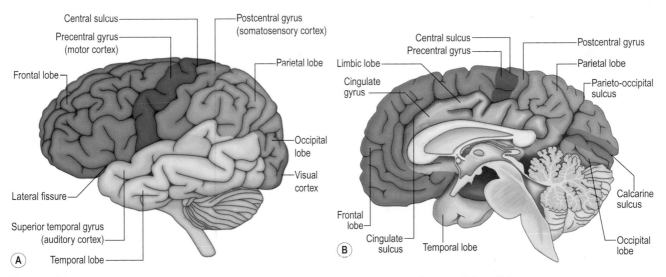

Figure 1.22 **Principal gyri, sulci and functional areas of the cerebral cortex. (A) Lateral aspect; (B) medial aspect.**

the medial surface, parietal and occipital lobes are separated by a deep **parieto-occipital sulcus**. On the medial aspect of the cerebral hemisphere, the **cingulate sulcus** runs parallel to the upper margin of the corpus callosum. This delineates a region of cortex that, together with parts of the medial aspect of the temporal cortex, is sometimes referred to as the **limbic lobe**.

The functions of the cerebral cortex are described in more detail in Chapter 13. It will be useful at the outset, however, to identify four important functional areas of cortex, one in each lobe (Fig 1.22).

- In the frontal lobe, the gyrus immediately in front of the central sulcus is referred to anatomically as the **precentral gyrus**. Functionally, this contains the **primary motor cortex**, which is the highest level in the brain for the control of movement. Here, in each hemisphere, the opposite half of the body is represented in a highly precise fashion.
- In the parietal lobe, facing the primary motor cortex across the central sulcus, lies the **postcentral gyrus** or **primary somatosensory cortex**. This is the site of termination of pathways carrying the modalities of touch,

pressure, pain and temperature from the opposite half of the body and it is the region where they are consciously perceived. The special senses have their highest level of representation in other areas.

- The **visual cortex** is located in the occipital lobe, mostly on the medial aspect of the hemisphere in the gyri above and below the horizontally orientated **calcarine sulcus**.
- In the temporal lobe lies the **auditory cortex**. It is localised to the **superior temporal gyrus**, which lies beneath, and parallel to, the lateral fissure.
- The limbic lobe is comprised primarily of the **cingulate gyrus**, lying on the medial aspect of the hemisphere, parallel to the corpus callosum, and the **hippocampal formation** and **amygdala** which lie within the temporal lobe. These complex structures are concerned with the emotional aspects of behaviour and with memory.

During development, the cerebral hemisphere takes on a C-shaped configuration as a result of the forward migration of the temporal lobe, such that the temporal pole comes to lie adjacent to the frontal lobe, separated from it by the lateral fissure. The lateral ventricle within the hemisphere, therefore, is also basically C-shaped with 'horns' extending into the frontal, occipital and temporal lobes (Fig. 1.18).

The basic structure of the cerebral hemisphere is an outer mantle of grey matter, the cerebral cortex, beneath which lies a large and complex mass of white matter consisting of nerve fibres running to and from the cortex (Figs 1.20, 1.21, 1.23).

Cortical afferent and efferent fibres which pass between the cerebral cortex and subcortical structures such as the corpus striatum, thalamus, brain stem and spinal cord are arranged in a characteristic radiating pattern, the **corona radiata**, which reaches out to the convolutions of the cortical surface (Fig. 1.23). Deeper inside the hemisphere the fibres are concentrated into a dense sheet of white matter, known as the **internal capsule** (Figs 1.20, 1.21, 1.23).

Deep inside the hemisphere, both medial and lateral to the internal capsule, lie additional masses of grey matter, often collectively referred to as the **basal ganglia**. The largest of these is the **corpus striatum**, which consists of the **caudate nucleus**, the **putamen** and the **globus pallidus** (Figs 1.20, 1.21). The caudate nucleus lies in the wall of the lateral ventricle throughout its extent and, like the ventricle, it is C-shaped. The basal ganglia are concerned with the control of muscle tone, posture and movement (Ch. 14).

Basic organisation of the brain

- The brain is conventionally divided into hindbrain, midbrain and forebrain.
- The hindbrain is further subdivided into the medulla oblongata, pons and cerebellum.
- The medulla, pons and midbrain constitute the brain stem.
- The forebrain consists of the diencephalon (thalamus and hypothalamus) and the cerebral hemisphere.
- Within the cerebral hemisphere lie several large nuclei called the basal ganglia or corpus striatum.
- The brain contains a system of cavities or ventricles containing CSF, which is produced by the choroid plexus.
- The brain possesses 12 pairs of cranial nerves, which carry afferent and efferent fibres.
- The two cerebral hemispheres are linked by the fibres of the corpus callosum.
- The surface of the cerebral hemisphere consists of cortical grey matter, which is folded to form gyri and sulci. Beneath the surface lie the dense fibre masses of the corona radiata and the internal capsule. The surface is divided into lobes:
  - Frontal lobe containing the primary motor and premotor cortices
  - Parietal lobe containing the primary somatosensory cortex
  - Temporal lobe containing the primary auditory cortex
  - Occipital lobe containing the primary visual cortex
  - Limbic lobe containing regions for memory and emotional aspects of behaviour.

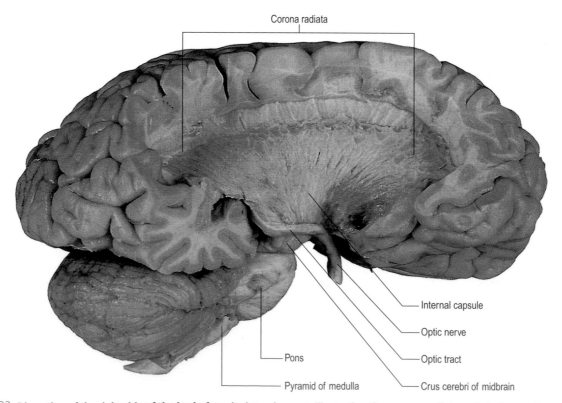

Corona radiata

Internal capsule

Optic nerve

Pons

Optic tract

Pyramid of medulla

Crus cerebri of midbrain

Figure 1.23 **Dissection of the right side of the brain from its lateral aspect, illustrating the corona radiata and the internal capsule.**

The major sensory pathways

Sensory information about the internal and external environment is carried to the CNS in afferent nerve fibres running in cranial and spinal nerves. Sensory information can be classified under the headings of 'special senses' and 'general senses'. The special senses are all carried in cranial nerves and are comprised of olfaction (cranial nerve I), vision (II), taste (VII and IX), and hearing and vestibular function (VIII). The special senses are dealt with in more detail elsewhere.

The general senses include the modalities of touch, pressure, pain and temperature (relayed from exteroceptors in the skin and interoceptors in the viscera), and awareness of posture and movement (from proprioceptors in joints, tendons and muscles). General sensory information from the trunk and limbs is carried in spinal nerves; from the head it is carried in the trigeminal nerve (cranial nerve V).

For all modalities in the category of general sensation, there is a sequence of three neurones between the sensory receptor located in the periphery and the perception of sensation at the level of the cerebral cortex (Fig. 1.24). The first neurone (**first-order neurone** or **primary afferent neurone**) enters the spinal cord, or the brain stem, through a spinal nerve, or the trigeminal nerve, on the same side of the body as its peripheral receptor is located. The cell body of the first-order neurone is located in the dorsal root

ganglion of a spinal nerve, or in the trigeminal ganglion. Within the CNS, the first-order neurone remains on the same side (ipsilateral) and synapses upon the second neurone (**second-order neurone**). The second-order neurone has its cell body in the spinal cord or brain stem, the exact location depending on the modality concerned. Its axon crosses over (decussates) to the other side of the CNS and ascends to the thalamus, where it terminates. The third neurone in the sequence (**third-order neurone**) has its cell body in the thalamus and its axon projects to the somatosensory cortex, located in the postcentral gyrus of the parietal lobe of the cerebral hemisphere.

More specifically, primary spinal afferents carrying coarse touch/pressure, pain and temperature information from the limbs and trunk terminate near their level of entry into the spinal cord. They synapse with second-order neurones, the axons of which decussate within a few segments and thereafter form the **spinothalamic tract**. In contrast, primary spinal afferents carrying proprioceptive information and discriminative (fine) touch ascend uninterrupted on the same side of the cord as their entry, forming the **dorsal columns** (fasciculus gracilis and fasciculus cuneatus). They terminate in the **dorsal column nuclei** (nuclei gracilis and cuneatus) located in the medulla. From here, second-order neurones decussate and ascend to the thalamus as the **medial lemniscus**. Primary afferent neurones that enter the brain stem in the trigeminal nerve terminate ipsilaterally

Figure 1.24 **Overview of the major pathways for general sensation.**

in the **trigeminal sensory nucleus**, one of the cranial nerve nuclei. From here, second-order neurones decussate and ascend to the thalamus as the **trigeminothalamic tract**. Second-order sensory neurones, of either spinal cord or brain stem origin, converge upon the same region of the thalamus (the ventral posterior nucleus), synapsing upon third-order neurones that project to the somatosensory cortex in the postcentral gyrus of the parietal lobe. Throughout the central projections of the somatosensory system there is a high degree of spatial segregation of the neurones representing different parts of the body (so-called **somatotopic** organisation). This is most dramatically demonstrated at the level of the cerebral cortex (see Fig. 13.20). Here the somatosensory area occupies a strip of cortex that extends from the medial aspect of the hemisphere (leg area) to the inferolateral aspect of the parietal lobe (head area).

The major motor pathways

The motor neurones that directly innervate skeletal muscle have cell bodies lying in the grey matter of the spinal cord and brain stem and are often referred to as **lower motor neurones**. They constitute the so-called 'final common pathway' by which the nervous system controls movement. In contrast, the neurones which control the activity of lower motor neurones are themselves collectively referred to as **upper motor neurones**. They form a number of **descending tracts** that run through the brain stem and spinal cord. Among the most important of these are the **corticospinal** and **corticobulbar tracts** (Fig. 1.25). These tracts originate partly from neurones in the motor area of the cerebral cortex, where the whole body is represented in a somatotopic fashion (Fig. 13.20). Axons pass through the internal capsule and into the brain stem, where most of them decussate to the other side. This means that movements of one side of the body are controlled by the opposite cerebral cortex. Corticobulbar fibres control the activity of motor neurones located in cranial nerve nuclei, which innervate skeletal muscles of the head and neck through the cranial nerves. Corticospinal fibres control the activity of motor neurones in the spinal cord, which innervate trunk and limb muscles. The place where corticospinal fibres cross over to the other side of the nervous system can be seen on the ventral aspect of the medulla (see Fig. 9.4) and is known as the **decussation of the pyramids**. Because of this, the corticospinal tract is also known as the **pyramidal tract**.

The main function of the corticobulbar and corticospinal pathways is the control of voluntary, skilled movements. A large proportion of the motor cortex and its descending pathways are, therefore, devoted to those parts of the body capable of delicate, so-called 'fractionated' movements, such

Figure 1.25 **Overview of the major motor pathways.**

as the muscles of speech and facial expression and the muscles controlling the hand.

Numerous brain structures apart from the corticospinal or pyramidal system are involved in the control of movement, posture and muscle tone; these are sometimes collectively known as **extrapyramidal** pathways. They include certain nuclei in the brain stem, such as the **vestibular nuclei** and the **reticular nuclei (reticular formation)**, and also the basal ganglia and related subcortical nuclei located in the forebrain. The vestibular and reticular nuclei influence spinal motor neurones through descending connections in the **vestibulospinal** and **reticulospinal tracts**. They are important in the control of muscle tone and the posture of the body. The basal ganglia exert their actions on the lower motor neurones of the brain stem and spinal cord of the contralateral side through complex, indirect pathways (Fig. 1.26). These include projections via the thalamus to the motor areas of the cerebral cortex and projections to the reticular formation of the brain stem. The basal ganglia are important in the facilitation of appropriate motor

behaviour and the inhibition of unwanted movements (Ch. 14).

The cerebellum is an important centre in which programmes of movement, generated in the motor region of the cerebral cortex, are compared with sensory feedback concerning the speed and direction of active movements of the limbs, head and neck in space. This is essential for accurate, coordinated, purposeful movement. The cerebellum receives afferent connections from the spinal cord *via* the **spinocerebellar tracts** and from the vestibular system and the motor cortex. Its efferent connections are complex but are primarily in the form of feedback to the thalamus and thence to the motor cortex (Fig. 1.27). Afferents to each side of the cerebellum come from the ipsilateral half of the spinal cord and brain stem and from the contralateral cerebral cortex. Efferent projections are directed to the contralateral thalamus and cerebral cortex through a decussation in the midbrain. Because of this and the decussation of cortical descending motor pathways, each side of the cerebellum coordinates the movements of the ipsilateral side of the body (Ch. 11).

Figure 1.26 **Overview of the connections of the basal ganglia.**

Figure 1.27 **Overview of the connections of the cerebellum.**

Basic clinical diagnostic principles

A knowledge of neuroanatomy is a prerequisite for the clinical diagnosis of disorders of the nervous system. The process of reaching a diagnosis proceeds by history-taking, then neurological examination and, finally, by confirmatory investigations (Fig. 1.28). History-taking provides clues to the aetiology or cause of disease, whereas the clinical examination pinpoints the site of the lesion (Fig. 1.29). A pathological lesion acting at a specific locality within the neuromuscular axis forms a recognisable syndrome, investigation of which leads to establishing the aetiology or diagnosis.

Aetiology of neurological disease

The disorders of the neuromuscular system are of four major types (Fig. 1.30) in relation to causation or aetiology.

For each major cause of disease there are appropriate types of investigation, leading to specific forms of treatment.

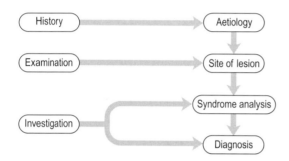

Figure 1.28 **The process of clinical diagnosis.**

Figure 1.29 **The central and peripheral nervous systems and possible sites of pathological lesion.**

Cause	Investigation/treatment
Extrinsic	Neurosurgery
Systemic	Medicine
Vascular	Cardiology
Intrinsic	Neurology

Figure 1.30 **The four major categories of disorders of the neuromuscular system.**

The four causes are ranked in order of clinical priority so that conditions that are common, potentially life-threatening, and reversible with prompt treatment, are either established or excluded first. Conditions that are rare, chronic and incurable can be considered later.

Extrinsic disorders

Extrinsic disorders lead to compression of the brain, spinal cord, nerve roots and peripheral nerves (Fig. 1.31) and are, therefore, surgically remediable. Investigations, such as the neuroradiological imaging of the central nervous system, must be promptly carried out prior to neurosurgical intervention. Delay in decompressive neurosurgery can lead to permanent paralysis, sensory loss and incontinence.

The cerebrum, spinal cord and peripheral nerves can be compressed by disease of adjacent structures. The brain may be compressed on its outer surface by blood clots (**haematomas**), abscesses and tumours arising within the skull and coverings of the cerebrum. Alternatively, the fluid-filled ventricles may compress the brain from within when blockage to the flow of CSF leads to a rise in pressure and expansion of the ventricles (**hydrocephalus**).

The spinal cord may be compressed by disease of the spine, such as arthritis (**spondylosis**), prolapsed intervertebral discs and bone tumours, as well as by tumours of the meninges (**meningiomas**). The central canal of the spinal cord, normally a minute vestigial space, may expand into a cavity (**syrinx**), compressing the nerve fibres in the centre of the cord (**syringomyelia**).

The cranial nerves emerging from the brain stem may be compressed, as they course through the cranium and leave the foramina of the skull, by tumours and swollen arteries (**aneurysms**). The spinal nerve roots leaving the spinal cord in the neck and back may be trapped by tumours and prolapsed intervertebral discs, causing pain, weakness and sensory loss in their region of distribution (**radiculopathy**). The peripheral nerves may become trapped at vulnerable pressure sites in the limbs by ribs and tough fibrous bands, leading to pain, weakness and sensory loss in their distribution (**entrapment neuropathy**).

Investigations for extrinsic disorders are chiefly neuroradiological (e.g. computed tomographic (CT) brain scan and magnetic resonance imaging (MRI)) to delineate the disorders (lesions) for neurosurgical decompression. Surgery may be required urgently to prevent permanent disability and that is why extrinsic disorders should be the first diagnostic consideration.

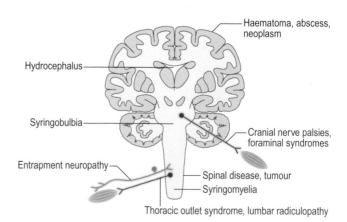

Figure 1.31 **Extrinsic disorders of the neuromuscular system.**

Systemic disorders

Systemic disorders are primarily disorders of organs other than the nervous system that disrupt neuromuscular function by abnormal metabolism (Fig. 1.32). The patient presents with a neurological condition or syndrome, but the cause lies primarily elsewhere. It may be intoxication with drugs (e.g. alcohol), dietary deficiency (e.g. of vitamin B), failure of the cardiorespiratory system, liver or kidneys, or hormonal (endocrine) disorders such as thyroid disease, diabetes mellitus and abnormalities in calcium and potassium balance. Investigations for systemic disease are chiefly haematological, biochemical tests and specific measures of cardiorespiratory, liver, renal and endocrine function. Treatment of the systemic disease by the appropriate specialist can lead to cure of the neurological disorder.

Vascular disorders

Vascular disorders (Fig. 1.33) damage the circulation to the nervous system in a number of ways:

- occlusion of the vessels (**thrombosis**)
- restriction of the blood and oxygen supply (**infarction**)
- bleeding into the nervous tissues (**haemorrhage**).

The rapid development of a vascular lesion is called a **stroke**. Congenital swellings of arteries (aneurysms) or tumours of blood vessels (**angiomas**) can compress cranial nerves and the brain itself. Investigations for vascular disorders are aimed at excluding abnormal clotting disorders of the circulating blood, testing the valves and muscles of the heart (echocardiography, electrocardiography and cardiac angiography), and displaying the vessels of the neck and brain by angiography. The treatment of vascular disorders may be haematological or cardiological and may require surgery to the heart or arteries in the neck and skull.

Intrinsic disorders

Intrinsic disorders (Fig. 1.34) are primary disorders of the nervous system itself. Intrinsic primary neurological disorders are uncommon and often chronic and irreversible, so that a more leisurely series of investigations can be chosen. Many nervous disorders are under genetic influences (**heredo-degeneration**). **Inborn errors of metabolism** lead to mental subnormality and disability in children and are usually caused by deficiencies of specific enzymes. **Paroxysmal disorders** consist of episodic loss of consciousness (**epilepsy**), excessive sleep (**narcolepsy**) and headache (**migraine**). **System degenerations** (Fig. 1.35) occur in youth and old age and lead to the premature death (**atrophy**) of certain neuromuscular components, with sparing of others. When

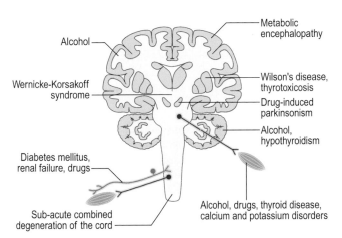

Figure 1.32 **Systemic disorders of the neuromuscular system.**

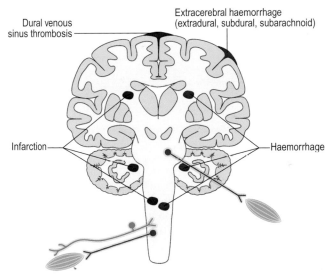

Figure 1.33 **Vascular disorders of the neuromuscular system.**

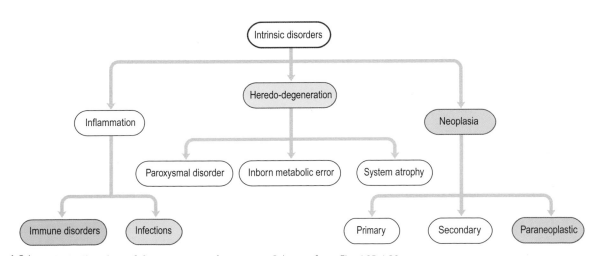

Figure 1.34 **Intrinsic disorders of the neuromuscular system.** Colours refer to Figs 1.35–1.39.

Figure 1.35 **Degenerative disorders of the neuromuscular system.**

Figure 1.37 **Paraneoplastic syndromes of the neuromuscular system.**

Figure 1.36 **Neoplasia of the neuromuscular system.**

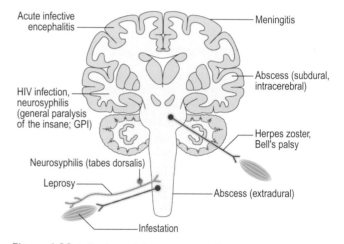

Figure 1.38 **Infections of the neuromuscular system.**

system degenerations occur in youth they often have an obvious hereditary or genetic cause: for example, the **muscular dystrophies**, the **hereditary sensorimotor neuropathies**, **hereditary spastic paraparesis**, **cerebellar ataxias** and **Huntington's disease**. When they occur later in life they are more often sporadic: e.g. **motor neurone disease**, **Parkinson's disease** and **Alzheimer's disease**. The system degenerations are remarkably selective; for example, in motor neurone disease there is paralysis of muscle but no abnormalities of sensation, whereas in Alzheimer's disease, there is severe amnesia but no paralysis.

Basic clinical diagnostic principles

- History-taking, clinical examination and investigations lead to the diagnosis of the cause (aetiology) of disease.
- The site of the lesion(s) determines the clinical syndrome revealed by the neurological examination.
- Disorders of the nervous system can be classified as extrinsic, systemic, vascular or intrinsic.
- Intrinsic disorders consist of system degenerations (atrophy), inborn errors of metabolism, paroxysmal disorders, neoplasms, infections and immune disorders.

Neoplasia refers to excessive, uncontrolled growth of tissues forming a benign or malignant tumour. Primary neoplasms arise in the neuromuscular tissues themselves (Fig. 1.36); secondary neoplasms spread in the circulation from other primary organ sites (e.g. lung or breast). Rarely, tumours at distant sites damage the nervous system by humoral or immune mechanisms and the resulting disorders are termed non-metastatic, or paraneoplastic, syndromes (Fig. 1.37).

Inflammation of neuromuscular tissue may result from **infection** by microorganisms (Fig. 1.38) and can affect different structures: e.g. the meninges (**meningococcal meningitis**), the brain (**viral encephalitis, neurosyphilis**) or peripheral nerves (**leprosy**). Alternatively, inflammation can occur in **immune disorders** (Fig. 1.39), in the absence of infection. The most common immune disorder of the CNS is **multiple sclerosis**. Immune disorders may also strike peripheral nerves (**acute inflammatory neuropathy** or the **Guillain–Barré syndrome**), the neuromuscular junction (**myasthenia gravis**) or muscle (**polymyositis**). Inflammatory disorders are investigated by microbiological and serological tests of the blood and CSF. Treatment of infection with antimicrobial agents and suppression of immune responses by drugs such as corticosteroids may cure or control these infective or immune diseases.

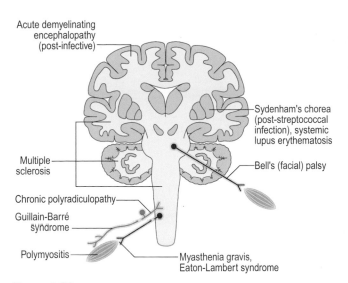

Figure 1.39 **Immune disorders of the neuromuscular system.**

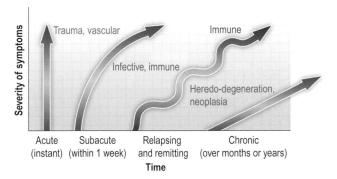

Figure 1.40 **History (onset) limits possible aetiologies.**

Time course of disease

History-taking can be valuable in suggesting the likely cause of illness by determining the rate of evolution of the disorder, which is often characteristic of the different aetiologies (Fig. 1.40). Disorders of sudden (acute), dramatic onset are caused by external injury (trauma) or a vascular accident (stroke). When the condition develops over days (subacute) to become maximal in about 1 week, this is strongly suggestive of an inflammatory disorder, which may be infective (e.g. meningitis) or immune (e.g. multiple sclerosis). Recovery from immune disorders takes weeks or months, or it is incomplete. Moreover, immune disorders often run a relapsing and remitting course, with acute events superimposed on chronic decline over the months and years. This paroxysmal course is highly characteristic of multiple sclerosis; hence the name of the disease. System degenerations, by contrast, take many years to develop (chronic) and the onset is often difficult to date, especially since patients accommodate slowly to their accumulating disability. In muscular dystrophy, hereditary sensorimotor neuropathies, and Parkinson's and Alzheimer's diseases, the disorders may last from 5 to 30 years. Neoplasms or tumours usually develop over months or years, with symptoms such as epileptic seizures and headache. Only rarely do highly malignant tumours (gliomas and secondary tumours) declare themselves over days or weeks.

Site of the lesion and clinical syndromes

Whatever the cause of a lesion may be, its site in the neuromuscular system leads to a characteristic syndrome. This is defined clinically by careful examination of the cranial nerves, the motor system, reflexes, sensation and coordination. In this book, the functional status of these systems is depicted diagrammatically (Fig. 1.41) so that the syndromes produced by particular types of lesion can be illustrated pictorially in a way that links neuroanatomy with clinical signs. In appropriate chapters, the description of the anatomy and basic functions of the nervous system is accompanied by figures, based upon the prototypical Figure 1.41, that summarise the principal clinical syndromes in terms of sensory and motor deficits. In order to understand fully the relationship between neuroanatomy and clinical signs it is necessary to know the routes of the major sensory and motor pathways, the significance of lesions of the 'lower motor neurone' and 'upper motor neurone', and the general functions of the cerebellum, basal ganglia and cerebral cortex.

The neuroanatomical information contained in this chapter represents the minimal and essential knowledge required before the clinical approach to the neurological patient. Without this knowledge, it is impossible to interpret the significance of the signs elicited on examination of the nervous system as described in the standard texts on 'clinical methods'. The continual practice of the examination of the nervous system through experience, and the development of clinical acumen, permit the highly accurate localisation of lesions within the central and peripheral nervous systems. The site of the lesion may be strictly focal – for example, a tumour in the left cerebral hemisphere, or may represent localisation within a functional neuroanatomical system – for example, the upper and lower motor neurones in motor neurone disease, or the peripheral nerves in sensorimotor polyneuropathy. A further delineation of focal lesions is to determine whether they lie within the nervous system (intrinsic lesions) or whether they lie outside and compress the nervous system (extrinsic lesions). This is an important distinction since extrinsic lesions represent disorders which are potentially remediable by neurosurgery.

There are certain principles which can be drawn from the organisation of the neuroanatomical structures described which are of high explanatory value to the clinician in determining the site of the lesion.

Major sensory pathways

Sensation in the trunk and limbs is conducted from sensory receptors in the periphery by the peripheral nerves and nerve roots to the dorsal root ganglia and then into the spinal cord. Within the spinal cord there is a divergence of sensory pathways carrying different sensory modalities (Fig. 1.24). The sensory pathways for pain and temperature decussate within the spinal cord and ascend in the contralateral spinothalamic tract to reach the thalamus and thence the contralateral sensory cortex of the cerebral hemisphere. In contrast, tactile and proprioceptive pathways ascend ipsilaterally in the dorsal (posterior) columns of the spinal cord before decussating in the lower brain stem and passing, via the thalamus, to the contralateral sensory cortex.

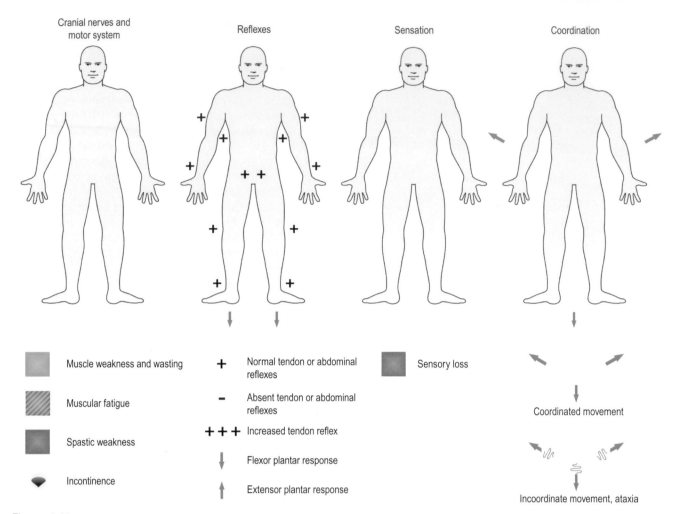

Figure 1.41 **Prototypical figure for illustration of major syndromes of the neuromuscular system.** Throughout the text, simplified outlines of the major anatomical–clinical syndromes are presented diagrammatically following the conventional neurological examination of cranial nerves, motor function, reflexes, sensation, coordination and mental state described in textbooks of clinical methods.

Patterns of sensory loss in disease

- Unilateral lesions of the spinal cord or lower brain stem lead to dissociated sensory loss.
- Lesions of the upper brain stem or cerebral hemisphere lead to loss of all sensation on the contralateral side of the body.

This divergent arrangement permits lesions of the spinal cord and brain stem to damage one pathway preferentially and spare the other. The term **dissociated sensory loss** refers to the clinical finding of selective loss of the modalities of touch and proprioception, with preservation of pain and temperature modalities, or *vice versa*. This selective loss of sensory modalities results from the selective involvement by lesions of the functionally specific pathways for touch/proprioception or pain/temperature. Lesion of the dorsal columns of the spinal cord leads to an ipsilateral loss of touch/proprioception below the level of the lesion. In contrast, lesion of the spinothalamic tract leads to contralateral loss of pain/temperature below the level of the lesion.

A unilateral lesion of the thoracic spinal cord, for example, leads to an ipsilateral loss of touch sensation and proprioception and a contralateral loss of pain and temperature sensation in the trunk and lower limbs below the level of the lesion. In addition, as described below, there is an ipsilateral 'pyramidal weakness' of the lower limb. Collectively, these are known as a hemicord or **Brown–Séquard syndrome** (see Fig. 8.21E).

Selective lesion in the brain stem of the medial lemniscus leads to loss of touch sensation, whereas lesion of the trigeminothalamic tract leads to loss of pain and temperature sensation in the face. Therefore, the clinical finding of dissociated sensory loss implies the presence of an intrinsic, focal lesion within the spinal cord or brain stem.

Because of the decussation of all ascending sensory pathways in either the spinal cord or lower brain stem, lesions of the upper brain stem or cerebral hemisphere lead to loss of all sensation on the opposite (contralateral) side of the body. (See also spinal cord lesions in Figs 8.21A–E, brain-stem lesions in Fig. 9.14 and unilateral cerebral hemisphere lesions in Fig. 13.19.)

Major motor pathways

The motor neurones arising in the brain stem and forming the cranial nerves, together with those leaving the ventral horns of the spinal cord in the motor roots of spinal nerves, are called lower motor neurones and they innervate specific muscle fibres. Damage to lower motor neurones leads, therefore, to weakness (**paresis**) or **paralysis** and **wasting** of individual muscles. The muscles show depressed deep tendon reflexes (**hyporeflexia**) and they lose their tone (**hypotonia**). Spontaneous contractions of the muscle fibres associated with a single motor nerve (motor unit) occur when the muscle fibres are denervated and are seen as **fasciculations**, i.e. ripple-like movements of muscle beneath the skin. Since all lower motor neurones innervate muscles on the same side of the body as the location of the nerve cell body, the effects of lower motor neurone lesions are seen ipsilateral to the lesion.

The descending motor pathways that control the activity of lower motor neurones are themselves referred to as upper motor neurones. They arise from the cerebral cortex and brain stem. The corticospinal (pyramidal) and corticobulbar pathways are particularly important (Fig. 1.25). These descending motor pathways are highly organised somatotopically but are also concerned with concerted movements of the limbs. Damage to the corticospinal pathway (upper motor neurone lesion) leads to loss of individual movements of the digits and a breakdown in movements of extension and abduction of the upper limbs and of flexion of the lower limbs. This characteristic weakness of movements is clinically referred to as a **pyramidal weakness**.

Lower and upper motor neurone lesions

Damage to lower motor neurones is associated with a number of motor signs and symptoms that distinguish it from upper motor neurone lesions. The distinction between lower and upper motor neurone syndromes is critical in neurological examination and diagnosis. The clinical signs of damage to the upper neurone functions are often referred to as pyramidal signs.

Lower motor neurone syndrome
- Weakness (paresis) or paralysis (plegia) of individual muscles
- Wasting of muscles
- Visible spontaneous contractions of motor units (fasciculation)
- Reduced resistance to passive stretching (hypotonia)
- Diminution or loss of deep tendon reflexes (hyporeflexia or areflexia).

Upper motor neurone syndrome
- Weakness or paralysis of specific movements (extension of the upper limbs and flexion of the lower limbs, termed 'pyramidal weakness')
- No wasting of muscles
- Increased resistance to passive stretching of muscles (spasticity); initial resistance to muscular stretching followed by relaxation (clasp-knife response)
- Hyperactivity of deep tendon reflexes (hyperreflexia)
- Emergence of the extensor plantar response (positive Babinski reflex) leading to dorsiflexion of the great toe on stimulation of the sole of the foot
- Loss of abdominal reflexes.

Pyramidal weakness is also associated clinically with overactive tendon stretch reflexes (**hyperreflexia**) and with increased muscle tone (**hypertonia**), i.e. resistance to passive limb movement, termed **spasticity**. The increase in tone occurs at the initial stretch of the limb muscles and is then followed by relaxation of tone (**clasp-knife response**). Spasticity manifests in the flexor muscles of the upper limbs and extensor muscles of the lower limbs. These are also the stronger muscle groups in the respective limbs, and the combination of spasticity and greater power contributes to the development of an abnormal posture in which the arms are relatively fixed in flexion and the legs in extension (see Fig. 13.19). The lower limb also demonstrates the positive **Babinski reflex** (dorsiflexion of the great toe on stimulation of the sole of the foot), which is considered as pathognomic of corticospinal tract damage.

The fact that the descending motor pathways in the corticobulbar and corticospinal tracts decussate in the lower brain stem means that a unilateral lesion in the cerebral hemisphere (see Fig. 13.19) or brain stem (see Fig. 9.14) leads to contralateral paralysis of the limbs.

The use of the term 'pyramidal' to describe the effects of upper motor neurone lesions implies that these clinical features result solely from damage to the pyramidal, or corticospinal, tract. However, individual tracts are rarely damaged in isolation and, therefore, it is often difficult to attribute clinical deficits to involvement of particular pathways. Damage to the pyramidal tract itself probably accounts for the loss of discrete movements and the appearance of the Babinski reflex. Hyperreflexia and spasticity are due to the additional involvement of other pathways.

Cerebellum

The plan of an intended movement is transmitted to the cerebellum from the motor parts of the cerebral cortex via the brain stem (Fig. 1.27). Once the specific movement takes place, afferent impulses from sensory receptors of the limbs, conveying information about the actual movement, flow through the peripheral nerves into the spinal cord and ascend in the spinocerebellar tracts, via the brain stem to the cerebellum. The cerebellum, therefore, is in a unique position to compare the intended with the actual movements of the limbs in space. When there is a discrepancy between these, the cerebellum is able to correct deviant movements. This is achieved by ascending pathways travelling via the thalamus to the motor cortex and thence through descending fibres passing to the brain stem and spinal cord. There are also direct cerebellar connections to the vestibular and reticular nuclei of the brain stem.

Lesions of the cerebellar pathways lead to a cerebellar syndrome comprised of incoordination of eye movements (**nystagmus**), speech (**dysarthria**), the upper limbs (**intention tremor**) and gait (**ataxia**), in the absence of weakness or loss of sensation (see Fig. 9.14). The symptoms and signs occur on the same side as (ipsilateral to) the lesion in the cerebellum.

The lesion interrupting the cerebellar pathways may lie in the cerebellum itself, the brain stem or the ascending spinocerebellar pathways in the spinal cord. Unilateral lesions of the cerebellum lead to ipsilateral loss of coordination. Similarly, a unilateral lesion of the brain stem inevitably destroys the cerebellar connections to the cerebral hemisphere and spinal cord and leads to ipsilateral incoordination and, as described above, a contralateral pyramidal weakness of the limbs.

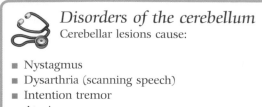

Disorders of the cerebellum
Cerebellar lesions cause:

- Nystagmus
- Dysarthria (scanning speech)
- Intention tremor
- Ataxia

The signs and symptoms occur ipsilateral to the lesion.

It is sometimes mistakenly thought that incoordination of the limbs is synonymous with a disorder of the cerebellum. This is not the case, whereas it is true that lesions of the cerebellum do lead to incoordination. A patient with a short leg and an arthritic hip joint, for example, will have an incoordinate gait. Moreover, weakness of the limbs due to disease of the central or peripheral nervous system will cause incoordination. Damage to the peripheral sensory nerves or to the dorsal columns of the spinal cord deprives the brain of proprioceptive information from the limbs, thus causing lack of coordination of the arms and an ataxic gait. This is known as 'sensory ataxia'. When patients with sensory ataxia close their eyes they readily lose their balance and this is known as **Romberg's sign**. This does not happen with lesions of the cerebellar pathways.

Because of these problems of interpretation it is conventional to carry out tasks of coordination at the end of the neurological examination in order to assess the contribution of orthopaedic deformities, neurological weakness and sensory loss to the degree of incoordination. If these prior deficits can be excluded on examination then incoordination can reliably be blamed on lesions of the cerebellar pathways themselves. This can sometimes be a difficult exercise; for example, in diseases such as multiple sclerosis, there are multiple lesions in the cerebellum, brain stem and spinal cord, each making a contribution to the nature and degree of neurological disability.

Basal ganglia
The basal ganglia, lying deep within the cerebral hemisphere, receive sensory and motor information from all parts of the cerebral cortex (Fig. 1.26) and also from the brain stem and spinal cord. Their functions are difficult to describe succinctly but they may be regarded as structures which facilitate useful, purposeful movements and inhibit unwanted movements. They are also important in the control of posture and muscle tone. These functions are illustrated by the symptoms of basal ganglia dysfunction, which cover a wide spectrum of manifestations. Lesions of the basal ganglia do not lead to loss of sensation, power or coordination. Instead, there is a loss of control of voluntary movement and posture, and changes in muscle tone. Unilateral lesions of the basal ganglia lead to a contralateral motor disorder.

One end of the spectrum of basal ganglia diseases is exemplified by **Parkinson's disease**. This is characterised primarily by slowness in the initiation and execution of movement (**akinesia**). There is also a characteristic slow, rhythmic **tremor** at rest. There is also increased muscular

tone (**hypertonia, rigidity**) of the limbs. Rigidity is characteristic of basal ganglia disorders and is manifest as resistance to passive movement throughout the whole excursion of the limb. It differs from spasticity, in which there is an initial resistance to passive movement of the limb, followed by relaxation (see above). In some forms of basal ganglia disease muscular tone is reduced (hypotonia).

The other end of the spectrum of basal ganglia diseases is exemplified by **Huntington's disease** and **levodopa-induced dyskinesia**. In these conditions there appear abnormal involuntary movements (**dyskinesias**) which take the form of inappropriate, quasi-purposeful fragments of normal movement (**chorea**). **Dystonia** is characterised by relatively fixed abnormal postures and may be associated with slow, serpentine twisting of the limbs (**athetosis**). In **Tourette's syndrome** there occur brief stereotypical repetitive movements, called **tics**. **Myoclonus** is characterised by sudden, shock-like muscle jerks, although its pathophysiology is often unrelated to the basal ganglia.

Disorders of the basal ganglia
Basal ganglia lesions cause:

- Slow initiation and execution of movement (akinesia)
- Increased muscular tone (rigidity)
- Abnormal involuntary movements (dyskinesias).

The signs and symptoms occur contralateral to the lesion.

Neuropsychological functions
The neuropsychological functions of language, perception, spatial analysis, learned skilled movements, memory and problem-solving (or executive functions) are organised within the cerebral hemispheres (Fig. 1.42). Accordingly, lesions of the brain stem, cerebellum and spinal cord are not accompanied by psychological deficits. The organisation of neuropsychological functions within the cerebral hemisphere is highly localised, as with the motor and sensory systems.

Language functions (speech, reading, writing and calculation) are organised in the regions of the frontal,

Figure 1.42 **Regional localisation of neuropsychological functions in the cerebral hemisphere and the syndromes associated with dysfunction.**

parietal and temporal lobes adjacent to the left lateral fissure, the so-called 'language area'. Whereas primary visual processes are organised in the occipital lobes, the perception or **recognition of objects** and human faces is organised in projections to the temporal lobes of the brain. The spatial ability to navigate the limbs and body in space (**visuospatial function**) is organised through projections to the parietal lobes. The premotor areas of the frontal lobes, including the supplementary motor area which lies on the medial aspect of the hemisphere, govern the enactment of learned, skilled movements of the head, neck and limbs (**praxis**). Structures in the medial aspects of the temporal lobes, part of the limbic system, are responsible for **learning** new information and recollecting from experience (**memory**). The organisation of behaviour involving problem-solving and the achievement of goal-directed behaviour (**executive function**) is organised within the prefrontal areas of the frontal lobes.

It can be deduced from these neuropsychological and anatomical correlations that lesions of the language area will lead to loss of speech (**aphasia**), reading (**alexia**), writing (**agraphia**) and calculation (**acalculia**), whereas lesions of the temporoparietal cortex lead to loss of perception (**agnosia**) and spatial orientation (**visuospatial disorientation**). Loss of the knowledge of learned skilled movements (**apraxia**) follows lesions of the premotor cortex. Bilateral disorders of the medial temporal lobes and limbic system lead to loss of memory function (**amnesia**). Damage to the prefrontal cortex leads to marked behavioural disturbance with loss of forethought, planning and appropriate affect, manifest in a marked change of personality and behaviour (**frontal lobe** or **dysexecutive syndrome**).

Investigation of neuromuscular disease

The clinical definition of a particular syndrome permits the choice of appropriate investigations to confirm the diagnosis. The major focus of investigations involves:

- CSF analysis
- neuroradiology
- neurophysiology
- neuropathology (biopsy).

Lumbar puncture enables the measurement of CSF pressure and the collection of CSF for bacteriological, biochemical, serological and cytological analyses. These may reveal the presence of blood (**subarachnoid haemorrhage**), infection, immune disease such as multiple sclerosis or the presence of tumour cells.

Neuroradiology encompasses a number of techniques that can be used to obtain both structural and functional images of the central nervous system and surrounding structures. Conventional **X-ray imaging** is applied to the skull and vertebral column, whilst structural images of the brain and spinal cord are obtained using **computed tomography** (**CT**; Fig. 1.43) and **magnetic resonance imaging** (**MRI**; Fig. 1.44). Functional images of regional cerebral blood flow, cerebral metabolism and the binding of ligands such as drugs to the brain can be obtained using **single photon emission computed tomography** (**SPECT**; Fig. 1.45) and **positron emission tomography** (**PET**). In contrast radiology, an opaque medium is injected into the arteries or veins (**angiography**) to delineate the blood vessels (Fig. 1.46).

| 1 | Frontal lobe | 3 | Brain stem |
| 2 | Caudate nucleus | 4 | Temporal lobe |

Figure 1.43 **Axial computed tomography (CT) scan of the head.**
(Courtesy of Professor P D Griffiths, Academic Unit of Radiology, University of Sheffield, Sheffield, UK).

1	Cerebral hemisphere	5	Medulla
2	Corpus callosum	6	Pons
3	Cerebellum	7	Midbrain
4	Spinal cord	8	Thalamus

Figure 1.44 **Sagittal magnetic resonance image (MRI) of the head.**
(Courtesy of Professor A Jackson, Wolfson Molecular Imaging Centre, University of Manchester, Manchester, UK.)

1 Frontal lobe
2 Striatum
3 Occipital lobe

Figure 1.45 **Axial single photon emission computed tomography (SPECT) scan of the head in a normal subject.** The radiolabelled ligand ^{123}I-FP-CIT has been used to label the dopamine transporter (DAT) in the striatum. (Courtesy of Professor D J Brooks, Faculty of Medicine, Imperial College, London, UK.)

1 Anterior cerebral artery
2 Middle cerebral artery
3 Ophthalmic artery
4 Left internal carotid artery

Figure 1.46 **Lateral view of a carotid angiogram.** This image was obtained by injecting an iodine containing contrast agent selectively into the left internal carotid artery. This was done via a catheter that was introduced into the femoral artery and then guided into the aortic arch and carotid artery under fluoroscopic control. (Courtesy of Professor P D Griffiths, Academic Unit of Radiology, University of Sheffield, Sheffield, UK.)

Neurophysiology addresses the electrical activity of the CNS by **electroencephalography (EEG)** and the detection and measurement of **evoked responses** to visual, auditory and somatosensory stimuli. **Central magnetic stimulation** to the brain enables measurement of the motor conduction time to the spinal cord and limb muscles. In the peripheral nervous system, measures of motor and sensory **nerve conduction velocity** and **evoked sensory action potentials** are combined with measurement of individual muscle responses to voluntary and electrically evoked contraction (**electromyography**).

The **biopsy** of nerve, muscle and brain tissue sheds light on the pathophysiological process (e.g. axonal degeneration, demyelination, muscular degeneration) and on the aetiology (e.g. inflammation, neoplasia).

Chapter 2
Cells of the nervous system

The principal functional unit of the nervous system is the nerve cell or neurone. These cells are highly specialised for the encoding, conduction and transmission of information. Neuroglial cells, or glia, are present in the nervous system in even larger numbers than neurones. Glia do not take part directly in information processing but are, nonetheless, crucial for normal neural function. Other cells are also present in the nervous system, such as those forming the walls of blood vessels but, unlike neurones and neuroglia, these are not unique to the nervous system.

The neurone

Neuronal structure

The main structural features, common to all neurones, have been described briefly in Chapter 1. There are, however, numerous variations on the basic plan. The size of the cell body varies considerably, depending upon location and function. For example, some interneurones in the CNS have cell bodies as small as 5 μm in diameter, while the cell bodies of motor neurones innervating striated muscle may exceed 100 μm. The size of the cell body is usually correlated with the length of the axon. Therefore, small interneurones usually have short axons, perhaps only a fraction of a millimetre in length. At the other extreme, large motor neurones possess long axons (e.g. those passing from the spinal cord to the muscles of the foot have axons about 1 m in length).

The **dendritic arborisation** of neurones also shows great variation in the number, size and density of branches, which reflects the organisation of afferent inputs to the cell. For example, pyramidal cells in the cerebral cortex have one or two apical dendrites which course towards the pial surface (Fig. 2.1A) while Purkinje cells in the cerebellar cortex have highly complex, tree-like dendritic arborisations (Fig. 2.1B).

The configuration of the cell body in relation to the dendrites and axon follows one of three basic patterns (Fig. 2.2). **Multipolar** neurones are by far the most common. Typically, they possess an axon and a number of dendrites that arise directly from the cell body. **Bipolar** neurones

have a centrally placed cell body, from which extend a single dendrite and a single axon. Bipolar neurones occur in the afferent pathways of the visual, auditory and vestibular systems. **Unipolar** neurones possess a single process emerging from the cell body. This divides into dendritic and axonal branches. Neurones of this type constitute the primary afferents of spinal and some cranial nerves, having their cell bodies in the dorsal root ganglia and sensory ganglia of cranial nerves.

Like most other cells, neurones possess a nucleus. This is usually located in the centre of the cell body and contains the chromosomal DNA. The rest of the intracellular space is occupied by cytoplasm, which contains numerous organelles and inclusions (Fig. 2.3). Many of these are common to cells other than neurones, but some have particular prominence or significance in neurones. Numerous microscopic clumps of **Nissl granules** (bodies, substance) can usually be seen in nerve cell bodies stained with basophilic dyes. Nissl granules consist of rough endoplasmic reticulum and associated ribosomes. The ribosomes contain RNA (which accounts for the basophilic staining properties) and are the sites of protein synthesis. Nerve cells are highly metabolically active and, therefore, the Nissl granules are often very prominent (Fig. 2.4).

Neurones contain a complex meshwork of structural protein strands called **neurofilaments**, which are assembled into larger **neurofibrils** (Fig. 2.3). They also possess a system of **neurotubules** that are involved in the transport of materials throughout the cell. Transport of materials occurs both away from and towards the cell body (**anterograde** and **retrograde transport**, respectively). This phenomenon is exploited in experimental neuroanatomical tracing techniques.

Some neurones contain pigment granules. **Neuromelanin** is a brown-black pigment produced as a by-product of the synthesis of catecholamines. Neuromelanin thus occurs most abundantly in cell groups that utilise catecholamines as their neurotransmitter, notably the pars compacta of the substantia nigra in the midbrain and the locus coeruleus in the pons. **Lipofuscin** is a yellow-brown pigment that accumulates in some neurones with age.

Each nerve cell is a separate physical entity with a limiting cell membrane. In order for information processing to occur in networks of neurones, therefore, information has to pass between neurones. This occurs at synapses. The basic structure of the synapse has been outlined in Chapter 1. The most common location for synapse formation is between the terminal axonal arborisation of one neurone and the dendrite of another (**axodendritic** synapse). Other locations are also possible and they give **axosomatic**,

Figure 2.1 **(A) A pyramidal cell in the cerebral cortex (×100). (B) A Purkinje cell in the cerebellar cortex (×90) showing the diversity of dendritic arborisations.** (Golgi–Cox stain.)

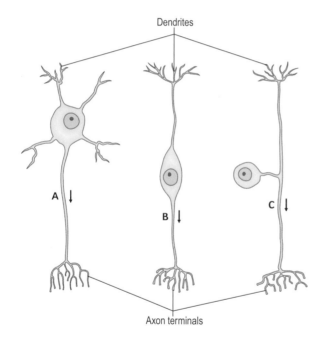

A   Multipolar
B   Bipolar
C   Unipolar

Figure 2.2 **Unipolar, bipolar and multipolar neurones.** Arrows indicate the direction of impulse conduction.

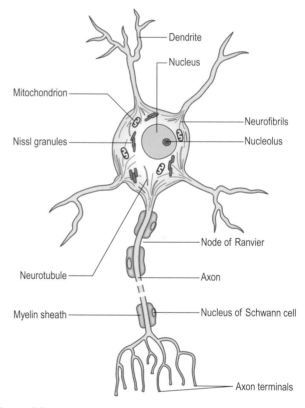

Figure 2.3 **A typical neurone.** The diagram illustrates the principal structural features, some intracellular organelles and the myelin sheath.

axoaxonal and **dendrodendritic** synapses. Neurotransmission between neurones occurs by release of specific chemical agents from the presynaptic ending that act upon receptors in the postsynaptic membrane.

Neurotransmitters

Neurotransmitter (transmitter) chemicals are stored in vesicles within the presynaptic ending. A single neurone is thought to release the same transmitter at all its synapses, and all neurones of a particular type, in terms of origin, termination and function, utilise the same transmitter.

Numerous transmitter substances have been identified at various sites in the nervous system. It has long been known that **acetylcholine** (ACh) is the transmitter between motor neurones and striated muscle. It is also the transmitter at autonomic ganglia and is released by postganglionic parasympathetic neurones. Some amino acids act as neurotransmitters. The most important are **glutamic acid** (glutamate) and **gamma-aminobutyric acid** (GABA) which occur widely and are the principal excitatory and

Figure 2.4 **A spinal motor neurone cell body.** Cresyl violet (a basophilic dye) stain shows prominent Nissl granules (×600).

Figure 2.5 **An astrocyte showing a process forming a perivascular endfoot on a blood capillary.** Cajal's gold chloride stain (×180).

inhibitory transmitters, respectively, in the CNS. Several monoamines are important transmitters. **Noradrenaline (norepinephrine)** is released by postganglionic sympathetic neurones peripherally as well as at some sites within the CNS. **Dopamine** and **serotonin (5-hydroxytryptamine, 5-HT)** also act as transmitters in the brain and spinal cord.

The effect of the neurotransmitter must be terminated once it has acted upon the postsynaptic membrane. This is achieved either by enzymic destruction of the transmitter or by its re-uptake into nerve endings and glia. For example, at the neuromuscular junction (see Fig. 3.6) and those neurone/neurone synapses where acetylcholine acts as transmitter, its action is terminated by the enzyme **acetylcholinesterase (AChE)**. In contrast, monoamine- and amino acid-mediated transmission are usually terminated by a re-uptake mechanism.

A number of peptides (neuropeptides) are stored and released at synapses. These include **enkephalin, substance P, cholecystokinin, somatostatin, dynorphin** and others. These peptides are often found co localised in the same neurones as amino acid or monoamine neurotransmitters and are sometimes called co-transmitters. It is believed that the neuropeptides modulate the release, re-uptake and postsynaptic effects of other transmitters and they are, therefore, often referred to as **neuromodulators**.

The neurone

- The neurone is the principal functional unit of the nervous system, specialised for the receipt, processing and transmission of information.
- Great variability exists in the size and shape of nerve cell bodies, their dendritic arborisations and axons, which reflects their functional specialisation.
- Nerve cells contain a number of organelles and inclusions. Among these are Nissl granules, neurofilaments and neurotubules, and pigment granules.
- A large number of neurotransmitter substances are known that mediate transmission between neurones. These include primarily acetylcholine, various amino acids (GABA, glutamate) and monoamines (dopamine, noradrenaline (norepinephrine) and serotonin).
- Peptide neuromodulators are co-localised with other transmitters in many neurones.

Neuroglia

Neuroglia are not directly involved in information processing but they are crucial for normal functioning of the nervous system. Various types of neuroglial cell are recognised: principally astrocytes, oligodendrocytes (oligodendroglia) and microglia.

Astrocytes

Astrocytes possess numerous processes. Some of these form so-called 'perivascular endfeet' upon the walls of blood capillaries (Fig. 2.5). Astrocytes are probably involved in the exchange of chemicals between the circulatory system and nervous tissue. It has been suggested that they constitute the **'blood–brain barrier'**, which restricts the access of circulating chemicals to the brain and spinal cord.

Oligodendrocytes

Oligodendrocytes possess few processes. Their main role is production of the myelin sheath that surrounds many axons in the CNS. **Schwann cells** perform this function in the peripheral nervous system. At any point along the length of a myelinated axon the myelin sheath is comprised of numerous concentric layers of the cell membrane of a single oligodendrocyte or Schwann cell (Fig. 2.6A). Each glial cell produces the myelin sheath over only a short segment of axon (up to about 1 mm). A long axon is, therefore, enveloped by the membranes of many glial cells. Adjacent segments of myelin, derived from different glial cells, are separated by a small gap, the **node of Ranvier** (Fig. 2.3). Unmyelinated axons also have a close association with glial cells but several axons usually share a single glial cell (Fig. 2.6B).

In myelinated axons, ionic fluxes across the axonal membrane, which mediate generation of the action potential, occur only at the nodes of Ranvier where the axon is exposed to the extracellular space. Between nodes, where the axon is insulated by myelin, depolarisation spreads by passive means (electrotonus). This mode of propagation of action potentials in myelinated axons is known as **saltatory conduction** (Latin: *saltare*, to jump), since the action potential may be thought of as 'jumping' from node to node. It is considerably faster than conduction in unmyelinated axons.

Figure 2.6 **(A) Transverse section through a myelinated axon, illustrating the structure of the myelin sheath. (B) Unmyelinated axons.**

Neuronal and glial disorders

Once development has been completed, individual neurones no longer replicate, but they do undergo continual repair to maintain their integrity. Hence, they are prone to **neurodegenerative diseases**, which in childhood and youth are often genetically determined and in the elderly are sporadic. Glia, unlike neurones, are capable of replication and they are, therefore, susceptible to neoplasia. Consequently, most brain tumours are gliomas and not tumours of neurones themselves. According to the cell of origin, they may become either **oligodendrogliomas** or **astrocytomas**. Microglia form part of the immune system and may proliferate to become cerebral **lymphomas**.

Multiple sclerosis

The myelin sheath of neuronal axons can be the seat of inflammatory diseases. In Europe and North America, the most common immune disorder of the CNS is multiple sclerosis, which leads to episodes of **demyelination** and **remyelination** of axons, corresponding to relapses and remission of neurological signs and symptoms. Since the disorder is chiefly of axons, not cell bodies, magnetic resonance (MR) brain imaging can detect abnormal signals from demyelinating foci in the cerebral white matter.

Microglia

Microglia are small cells with few processes. Microglia increase in number at sites of damage in the CNS and have a phagocytic role, similar to macrophages elsewhere. The **ependyma** consists of epithelial cells, which line the ventricles and cover the choroid plexus.

Neuroglia

- Neuroglia are important for normal neural function because of their ancillary roles.
- Astrocytes possess long processes that form perivascular endfeet around blood capillaries. They are involved in the transfer of materials between the vascular system and neural tissue.
- Oligodendroglia give rise to the myelin sheath surrounding axons in the CNS. Schwann cells form myelin in the peripheral nervous system.
- Microglia have a phagocytic role in injury to the nervous system.

Chapter 3
Peripheral nervous system

The peripheral nervous system consists of nerve endings, peripheral nerve trunks, plexuses and ganglia which link the CNS with other parts of the body. Most of the neurones in the peripheral nervous system are, therefore, either afferent or efferent with respect to the CNS.

- *Nerve endings* include sensory receptors, which detect changes in the internal and external environments, and efferent endings, which control the contraction of muscles and the activity of secretory glands.
- *Peripheral nerves* consist of spinal and cranial nerves and their branches, and the numerous named nerves to which these give rise.
- *Plexuses* (e.g. the brachial plexus and lumbosacral plexus) are structures in which fibres within certain spinal and cranial nerves are redistributed, without synapse, to form other peripheral nerves.
- *Peripheral ganglia* (e.g. dorsal root ganglia and autonomic ganglia) are structures outside the CNS where some nerve cell bodies are located.

Muscle

All behaviour depends on the ability to control the activity of skeletal muscles, which maintain posture and permit movement. Such control is subserved by a rich innervation of muscle with both motor and sensory neurones. Individual muscle cells (fibres) run parallel to the main axis of the muscle and fall into two main functional groups, namely **extrafusal** and **intrafusal** (Fig. 3.1).

Extrafusal muscle cells are by far the more numerous, constituting the bulk of the muscle and conferring its contractile strength. Extrafusal muscle fibres are innervated by **alpha motor neurones**, the cell bodies of which lie in the ventral horn of the spinal cord grey matter and in the motor cranial nerve nuclei of the brain stem. The axon of an individual alpha motor neurone typically branches within the target muscle to innervate a number of muscle fibres; the combination of a single motor neurone and the muscle fibres that it innervates is known as a **motor unit**. Motor units consist of relatively small numbers of muscle fibres in those muscles with which delicate, precise

Figure 3.1 **(A,B) Transverse sections through striated muscles showing extrafusal muscle fibres and intrafusal muscle fibres (within muscle spindles).**

movements can be made, such as the muscles of the hand and the extraocular muscles. In contrast, the motor units of large postural muscles – such as the quadriceps, for example – are comprised of relatively larger numbers of muscle cells. Intrafusal muscle fibres are highly specialised cells that act as sensory receptors. They occur in groups known as **muscle spindles**. Intrafusal muscle fibres bear sensory endings that signal muscle stretch and tension to the CNS. They also receive a motor innervation from

gamma motor neurones, whose cells of origin, like those of alpha motor neurones, lie in the ventral horn of the spinal cord and the motor cranial nerve nuclei of the brain stem. Gamma motor neurones function to control the sensitivity of the sensory endings.

🩺 *Myopathies*

- **Myopathy** is characterised by weakness and muscle wasting (of facial, bulbar and proximal limb muscles) with preservation of tendon reflexes and sensation (Fig. 3.2).
- **Polymyositis** is an immune disorder of muscle causing a painful or painless myopathy. When it occurs in the elderly, there is often a primary neoplasm elsewhere (paraneoplastic syndrome). In children, the skin is also inflamed, causing a rash. This is referred to as dermatomyositis.
- **Duchenne muscular dystrophy** is an inherited degenerative disorder of male children (X-linked inheritance). After 2–3 years of age, the child develops progressive weakness of the arms and legs with muscular contractures. He is wheelchair-bound by the age of 10 years and dies in youth.

Nerve endings

There are various, overlapping, conventions for the classification of nerve endings. Overall, they may be classified as either afferent or efferent. Afferent nerve endings respond to mechanical, thermal or chemical stimulation (mechanoreceptors, thermoreceptors or chemoreceptors, respectively). The nerve fibres to which they belong conduct action potentials to the CNS. If the afferent information reaches a conscious level then the pathway is termed sensory. Efferent (effector) nerve endings innervate muscle or secretory cells and, under control from the CNS, influence muscular contraction or cellular secretion. Nerve endings that induce movement are called motor; those that induce secretion are sometimes called secretomotor.

Afferent nerve endings

The sensory systems, or modalities, are broadly divided into the general and the special senses. The special senses are olfaction, vision, hearing, balance and taste and these are considered elsewhere.

There are three types of general sensory ending:

- **Exteroceptors.** These occur superficially in the skin and respond to nociceptive (painful) stimuli, temperature, touch and pressure.
- **Interoceptors.** These occur in viscera and respond principally to mechanical and chemical stimuli.
- **Proprioceptors.** These occur in muscles, joints and tendons and provide awareness of posture and movement (kinaesthesia).

Structurally, sensory nerve endings may be either unencapsulated or encapsulated (Fig. 3.3). Unencapsulated endings, or **free nerve endings**, consist of the terminal branches of sensory nerve fibres lying freely in the innervated tissue. These are the most abundant type of sensory ending, occurring widely in the integument and also within muscles, joints, viscera and other structures. In the skin, they mediate thermal and painful sensations. The parent nerve fibres are designated physiologically as group Aδ (III) finely myelinated and group C unmyelinated fibres. These are of relatively

Figure 3.2 **Myopathy.**

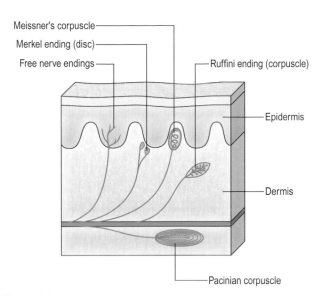

Meissner's corpuscle

Merkel ending (disc)

Free nerve endings

Ruffini ending (corpuscle)

Epidermis

Dermis

Pacinian corpuscle

Figure 3.3 **Sensory nerve endings in skin.**

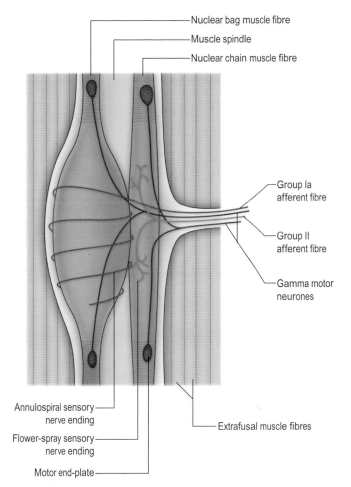

Nuclear bag muscle fibre

Muscle spindle

Nuclear chain muscle fibre

Group Ia afferent fibre

Group II afferent fibre

Gamma motor neurones

Annulospiral sensory nerve ending

Flower-spray sensory nerve ending

Motor end-plate

Extrafusal muscle fibres

Figure 3.4 **Innervation of intrafusal muscle fibres.** For clarity, only an annulospiral ending is shown on the nuclear bag fibre and only a flower-spray ending on the nuclear chain fibre although, in reality, both types of ending are found on both types of intrafusal fibre.

small diameter and slow conducting. **Merkel endings** (discs) are located near the border of the epidermis. These are slowly adapting receptors that respond to touch/pressure. The axons of origin are large and myelinated.

Encapsulated nerve endings are surrounded by a structural specialisation of non-neural tissue, the combination of nerve and its encapsulation often being referred to as a corpuscle. **Meissner's corpuscles** occur in the dermal papillae of the skin and are especially numerous in the fingertips. They respond with great sensitivity to touch. They are rapidly adapting receptors and are responsible for fine, or discriminative, touch. **Pacinian corpuscles** occur in skin and in deep tissues, e.g. surrounding joints and in mesentery. The largest are a few mm long and they are associated with group Aα (I) large diameter, myelinated axons. Pacinian corpuscles are rapidly adapting and respond to mechanical distortion, especially vibration. **Ruffini endings** (corpuscles) are slowly adapting mechanoreceptors occurring in the dermis of the skin.

Within skeletal muscles, intrafusal muscle fibres, which in small groups constitute muscle spindles, act as stretch receptors (Fig. 3.4). There are two types of intrafusal muscle fibre, referred to as **nuclear bag** and **nuclear chain** fibres. Intrafusal muscle fibres bear two types of sensory ending, which become activated when the muscle in which they lie is stretched. **Annulospiral** endings (Fig. 3.5) are associated with fast conducting group Ia afferent fibres and **flower-spray** endings are associated with slower conducting group II afferents. Muscle spindles are particularly abundant in muscles capable of fine, skilled movements. They are important in kinaesthesia and in the control of muscle tone, posture and movement. Their functional importance in motor control is considered in more detail in Chapter 8.

Golgi tendon organs occur in tendons and respond to tension.

Efferent nerve endings

Efferent endings occur in association with muscle and secretory cells. The endings resemble the synapses that occur between neurones. Transmission is by chemical means, depolarisation of the endings causing release of a neurotransmitter that acts upon receptors in the target cell membrane. In striated muscle, both alpha motor neurones (innervating extrafusal muscle fibres) and gamma motor

Annulospiral nerve ending

Ia afferent nerve fibre

Figure 3.5 **An annulospiral nerve ending on intrafusal muscle fibre.**

neurones (innervating intrafusal muscle fibres) end upon muscle cells in synaptic specialisations called **neuromuscular junctions** or **motor end-plates** (Figs 3.6, 3.7). The neurotransmitter at all neuomuscular junctions in striated muscle is acetylcholine.

Nerve endings

- The peripheral nervous system consists of nerve endings, peripheral nerves, plexuses and ganglia.
- Nerve endings are broadly classified as afferent (sensory) or efferent (motor).
- Sensory endings function as mechanoreceptors, thermoreceptors or chemoreceptors.
- In terms of location, they can be subdivided into exteroceptors, interoceptors and proprioceptors.
- Structurally, they may consist of unencapsulated (free) nerve endings, or encapsulated endings (such as Meissner's and Pacinian corpuscles).
- Skeletal muscles contain muscle spindles, which are composed of intrafusal muscle fibres. These consist of nuclear bag and nuclear chain types. They possess annulospiral and flower-spray sensory endings.
- Efferent nerve endings are either motor end-plates in muscle or endings in association with secretory cells (secretomotor).
- Alpha motor neurones innervate extrafusal muscle fibres and gamma motor neurones innervate intrafusal muscle fibres.

Disorders of neuromuscular junction

Myasthenia gravis is an immune disorder; it is the most common disorder of the peripheral neuromuscular junction. It causes weakness and fatigue of cranial muscles (e.g. extraocular, facial and bulbar muscles) and limb (especially proximal) muscles. This occurs without muscular wasting, changes in reflexes or sensation (Fig. 3.8). Treatment with drugs that inhibit acetylcholine esterase (anticholinesterases) potentiates neuromuscular transmission, with relief of symptoms. Intravenous edrophonium (an anticholinesterase; Tensilon) is a diagnostic test for the disease and produces rapid, but brief, return of muscular power. The **Eaton–Lambert syndrome** causes similar fatigue but is a paraneoplastic syndrome and does not respond to anticholinesterases.

Peripheral nerves

The term peripheral nerve applies to all the nerve trunks and branches that lie outside the CNS. They are the principal route through which the brain and spinal cord communicate with the rest of the body. A typical peripheral nerve consists of numerous nerve fibres, which may be either afferent or efferent with respect to the CNS.

Some peripheral nerve fibres are myelinated; others are unmyelinated. Within peripheral nerves, the nerve fibres are arranged in bundles and surrounded by sheaths of connective tissue (Fig. 3.9). Between individual fibres is a delicate connective tissue known as **endoneurium**. Bundles of fibres are surrounded by **perineurium** and the whole nerve is ensheathed by a tough coat known as **epineurium**.

Figure 3.6 **Motor end-plates on extrafusal muscle fibres in striated muscle. (A)** Ranvier's gold chloride stain showing efferent nerve fibres terminating in neuromuscular junctions (×600); **(B)** Acetylcholine esterase stain. The neurotransmitter at the neuromuscular junction is acetylcholine. The action of the transmitter is terminated by the enzyme acetylcholine esterase. The brown stain shows the specific localisation of the enzyme at the neuromuscular junction (×500).

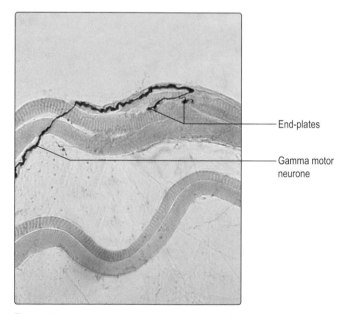

End-plates

Gamma motor neurone

Figure 3.7 **A gamma motor neurone ending in a motor end-plate on an intrafusal muscle fibre.**

This configuration provides strength and support for the nerve. The cranial and spinal meninges are continuous with the connective tissue sheaths of spinal and cranial nerves. Thus, the dura mater is continuous with the epineurium, while the arachnoid and pia are continuous with the perineurium and endoneurium.

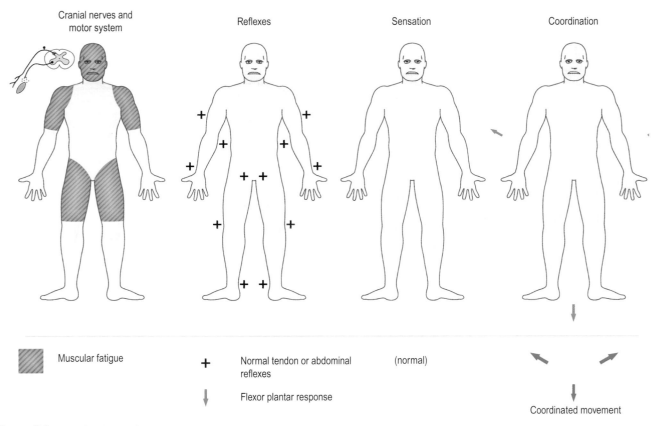

Cranial nerves and motor system | Reflexes | Sensation | Coordination

	Muscular fatigue
+	Normal tendon or abdominal reflexes
↓	Flexor plantar response
	(normal)
	Coordinated movement

Figure 3.8 **Myasthenia gravis.**

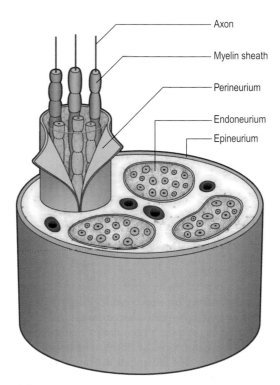

- Axon
- Myelin sheath
- Perineurium
- Endoneurium
- Epineurium

Figure 3.9 **The structure of a peripheral nerve.**

Degeneration and regeneration

When a peripheral nerve fibre is transected or otherwise seriously damaged, the portion distal to the transection (furthest from the cell body) undergoes degeneration and dies. This is known as **anterograde** or **Wallerian degeneration**. The proximal portion of the neurone, which remains attached to the cell body, may, however, survive and eventually undergo recovery or **regeneration**. The further from the cell body that transection occurs, the more likely it is that the cell body will survive. Initially, it too usually shows degenerative changes, known as **retrograde degeneration**. This is characterised by dispersal and loss of staining of Nissl granules (chromatolysis), swelling of the cell body and movement of the normally central nucleus to a peripheral location. If the cell recovers, the distal end of the surviving nerve fibre undergoes sprouting. If the two ends of the peripheral nerve are physically aligned (e.g. by surgery following traumatic injury), the new regenerating fibres may enter the endoneurial tubes that have lost their nerve fibres. Continued growth of the new fibres, at a rate of 1–2 mm/day, may eventually lead to reinnervation of the original structure and recovery of function. Many factors influence the degree to which successful reinnervation and functional recovery take place.

The degenerative processes that follow nerve cell injury are essentially similar in the CNS. Sprouting of surviving neurones also occurs in the CNS, but the re-establishment of previous connections does not, unfortunately, take place to any significant extent.

a	Upper lateral cutaneous of arm	k	Ilioinguinal
b	Medial cutaneous of arm	l	Obturator
c	Lower lateral cutaneous of arm	m	Sapheneous
d	Lateral cutaneous of forearm	n	Lateral cutaneous of leg
e	Medial cutaneous of forearm	o	Superficial peroneal (musculocutaneous)
f	Radial	p	Deep peroneal
g	Median	q	Posterior cutaneous of forearm
h	Ulnar	r	Posterior cutaneous of thigh
i	Lateral cutaneous of thigh	s	Medial cutaneous of thigh
j	Medial and intermediate cutaneous of leg	t	Sural

Figure 3.14 **The cutaneous distribution of spinal nerves (dermatomes) and named peripheral nerves.** Axial lines are in bold.

Figure 3.15 **The segmental innervation of limb movements.**

Radial nerve

Sensory	Motor
	Finger extensors
	Thumb extensors and abductors
	Wrist extensors
	Brachioradialis

Figure 3.16 **Sensory and motor deficits in peripheral nerve lesions.**

Compression and entrapment neuropathies

Peripheral nerves are vulnerable to extrinsic compression (e.g. excessive pressure on a recumbent limb) and to chronic entrapment by normal or diseased anatomical structures adjacent to them. The most common examples are **radial nerve** compression in the spiral groove of the humerus, and chronic entrapment of the **ulnar nerve** at the elbow and of the **median nerve** at the wrist (carpal tunnel syndrome) in the upper limb. Entrapment of the **lateral cutaneous nerve of the thigh** and compression of the **common peroneal nerve** at the head of the fibula occur in the lower limb (Fig. 3.16).

Peripheral nerves

- Many of the nerve fibres in cranial and spinal nerves become rearranged as they course peripherally, passing through the brachial or lumbosacral plexuses, to emerge as named peripheral nerves.
- Peripheral nerves consist of variable numbers of bundles, or fascicles, of nerve fibres.
- The nerve fibres are ensheathed in three connective tissue coverings: endoneurium, perineurium and epineurium.
- The endoneurial tubes within which individual axons lie are important for successful regeneration and reinnervation by nerves following nerve injury.
- The area of skin supplied by a spinal nerve is called a dermatome.
- The group of muscles innervated by a spinal nerve is called a myotome.

Chapter 4
Autonomic nervous system

The term 'autonomic nervous system' is used to describe those nerve cells located within both the central and peripheral nervous systems that are concerned with the innervation and control of visceral organs, smooth muscle and secretory glands. The principal function of the autonomic nervous system is broadly described as maintenance, or homeostasis, of the internal environment. This is achieved by regulation of cardiovascular, respiratory, digestive, excretory and thermoregulatory mechanisms, which occurs automatically and with relatively little volitional control.

Autonomic afferent and efferent nerve fibres enter and leave the CNS through spinal and cranial nerves. Within the spinal cord and brain stem they establish interconnections through which autonomic reflexes are mediated. Afferent fibres also establish connections with ascending neurones through which conscious awareness of visceral functions is achieved. Changes in the internal and external environment, and emotional factors, profoundly influence autonomic activity, most notably via descending connections from the **hypothalamus**. Autonomic efferent neurones differ from those of the somatic nervous system in that, in the autonomic nervous system, there is a sequence of two neurones between the CNS and the innervated structure (Fig. 4.1). The synaptic connection between the two neurones is located peripherally in an **autonomic ganglion**. The first neurone is, thus, called the **preganglionic neurone** and its cell body is located in the spinal cord or brain stem. The second neurone is referred to as the **postganglionic neurone** and its cell body is located peripherally in an autonomic ganglion.

The efferent neurones of the autonomic nervous system fall into two distinct anatomical and functional divisions or systems: namely, **sympathetic** and **parasympathetic**. Many, although not all, structures that receive autonomic fibres are dually innervated by both sympathetic and parasympathetic systems. These exercise antagonistic effects upon the innervated structure (Table 4.1).

Sympathetic division

Preganglionic sympathetic neurones are located exclusively in the thoracic and upper two or three lumbar segments of the spinal cord (Fig. 4.2). They lie in the **lateral horn** of the spinal grey matter, which is, therefore, only present at these levels (see Figs 8.8, 8.9). Preganglionic axons leave the cord in the ventral nerve roots and join the spinal nerve. Postganglionic sympathetic neurones have their cell bodies in one of two locations: either the **sympathetic chain** of ganglia that lies alongside the vertebral column, or the plexuses (coeliac, superior mesenteric, inferior mesenteric) that surround the main branches of the abdominal aorta. In order to reach any of these locations, preganglionic axons in the spinal nerve enter the sympathetic chain. Ganglia of the sympathetic chain are linked to those spinal nerves which contain sympathetic outflow by two small nerves, the **rami communicantes** (Fig. 4.3). Preganglionic fibres pass into the chain via the white ramus communicantes, so called because the constituent fibres are myelinated.

Those fibres concerned with innervation of structures in the head and thorax terminate in synaptic contact with postganglionic cell bodies in the sympathetic chain. The postganglionic fibres return to the spinal nerve via the grey ramus communicantes, so called because the fibres are unmyelinated. Those preganglionic fibres concerned with innervation of pelvic and abdominal viscera pass uninterrupted through the sympathetic chain and travel to the plexuses where their corresponding postganglionic cells are located. The neurotransmitter released by preganglionic sympathetic neurones is acetylcholine. The transmitter of postganglionic sympathetic cells is generally noradrenaline (norepinephrine), although the cells innervating sweat glands are cholinergic. The adrenal medulla is an exceptional organ in that it is directly innervated by preganglionic sympathetic neurones.

The effects of sympathetic nervous system activity are most apparent under conditions of stress, excitement or fear and are classically referred to as the 'fight or flight' response. The heart rate and blood pressure are increased. The bronchi are dilated to increase airflow to and from the lungs. Vasodilatation in skeletal muscles allows the

Figure 4.1 Basic organisation of the autonomic nervous system into preganglionic and postganglionic neurones. In the sympathetic division **(A)**, ganglia constitute the sympathetic chain, lying near the vertebral column. Preganglionic neurones, therefore, have relatively short axons, while postganglionic fibres are relatively long. In the parasympathetic division **(B)**, ganglia are located close to the target organ. Consequently, preganglionic axons are long and postganglionic axons are short.

Table 4.1 **Functions of the autonomic nervous system**		
Structure	**Sympathetic effect**	**Parasympathetic effect**
Iris of eye	Dilates pupil	Constricts pupil
Ciliary muscle of eye	Relaxes	Contracts
Salivary glands	Reduces secretion	Increases secretion
Lacrimal gland	Reduces secretion	Increases secretion
Heart	Increases rate and force of contraction	Decreases rate and force of contraction
Bronchi	Dilates	Constricts
Gastrointestinal tract	Decreases motility	Increases motility
Sweat glands	Increases secretion	
Erector pili muscles	Contracts	

increased blood flow required for energetic activity, while gastrointestinal blood flow and motility are decreased. Metabolic changes occur, such as an increase in blood glucose, to support high energy utilisation and sweating occurs to increase heat loss.

Parasympathetic division

Preganglionic parasympathetic neurones are located in the brain stem and the spinal cord (Fig. 4.4). Within the brain stem, such cells lie in cranial nerve nuclei associated with the oculomotor, facial, glossopharyngeal and vagus nerves and provide innervation for structures of the head, thorax and abdomen. The parasympathetic components of these nerves are described in Chapter 10. Within the cord, preganglionic parasympathetic neurones lie in the second, third and fourth sacral segments and provide innervation for pelvic viscera. The cell bodies of postganglionic parasympathetic neurones lie in ganglia that are located close to the structure which they innervate. Within the alimentary canal, these neurones contribute to the myenteric (Auerbach's) and submucosal (Meissner's) plexuses.

These plexuses are also referred to as the 'enteric nervous system'. Such a concept has arisen because the plexuses additionally contain afferent neurones and interneurones. The rich local interconnections of these cells are capable of sustaining the motility of the gastrointestinal tract in the absence of input from the CNS. Furthermore, these cells cannot simply be equated with the parasympathetic nervous system as traditionally defined, since they are known also to receive synaptic input from postganglionic sympathetic neurones. The neurotransmitter released by both preganglionic and postganglionic parasympathetic neurones is acetylcholine.

Lesions of the sympathetic nervous system

Primary autonomic failure is a chronic degenerative disease of the nervous system and leads to fainting through failure to control the heart rate and blood pressure (**postural syncope**), incontinence of urine and bowel, and impotence.

Horner's syndrome refers to drooping of the eyelid (ptosis) and constriction of the pupil (miosis) caused by damage to the sympathetic nerves to the levator palpebrae superioris and the radial (pupillodilator) fibres of the iris. The sympathetic nerves may be damaged as they descend in the brain stem (by stroke or tumour) and the spinal cord (by an expanded cavity or syrinx), as they emerge in the first thoracic nerve root (by tumour of the apical lung) and as they ascend in the sympathetic plexus around the carotid arteries (by swelling of the arteries in a migrainous attack).

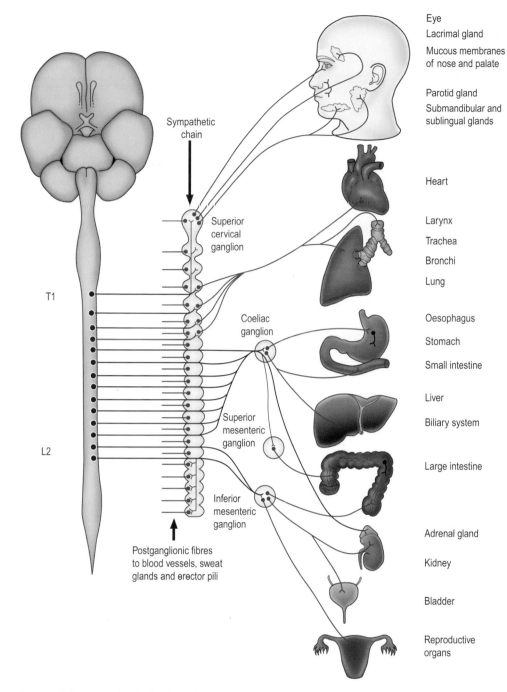

Eye
Lacrimal gland
Mucous membranes of nose and palate

Parotid gland
Submandibular and sublingual glands

Heart

Larynx
Trachea
Bronchi
Lung

Oesophagus
Stomach
Small intestine

Liver
Biliary system

Large intestine

Adrenal gland

Kidney

Bladder

Reproductive organs

Sympathetic chain

Superior cervical ganglion

T1

L2

Coeliac ganglion

Superior mesenteric ganglion

Inferior mesenteric ganglion

Postganglionic fibres to blood vessels, sweat glands and erector pili

Figure 4.2 **Organisation of the sympathetic division of the autonomic nervous system.**

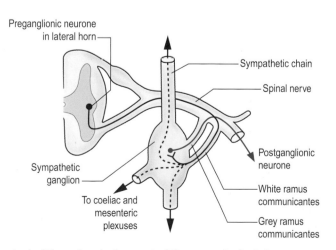

Preganglionic neurone in lateral horn

Sympathetic chain

Spinal nerve

Sympathetic ganglion

To coeliac and mesenteric plexuses

Postganglionic neurone

White ramus communicantes

Grey ramus communicantes

Figure 4.3 **Relationships between a typical thoracic spinal nerve and the sympathetic chain.**

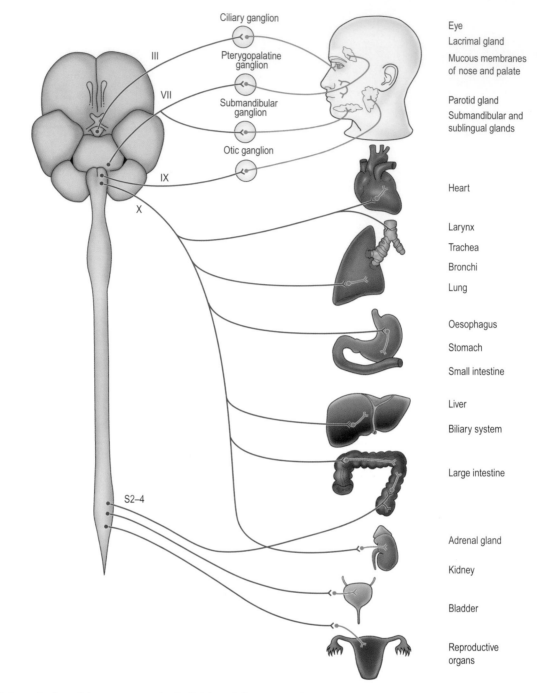

Figure 4.4 **Organisation of the parasympathetic division of the autonomic nervous system.**

Chapter 5
Coverings of the central nervous system

The CNS is supported and protected by bone and membranous coverings. The brain is located within the cranial cavity of the skull and the spinal cord lies in the vertebral, or spinal, canal within the vertebral column, or spine. Within their bony coverings, the brain and spinal cord are invested by three concentric membranous envelopes. The outermost membrane is the **dura mater**, the middle layer is the **arachnoid mater** and the innermost layer is the **pia mater**. The vertebral column and spinal meninges are described in Chapter 8; consequently, only the skull and cranial meninges are considered here.

Skull

The brain lies on the floor of the cranial cavity, which, together with the bones of the cranial vault, provides support and protection from physical injury. The floor of the cranial cavity consists of three **fossae**. Each of these accommodates particular parts of the brain and possesses **foramina** through which cranial nerves and blood vessels enter and leave the cranial cavity (Fig. 5.1).

Anterior cranial fossa

The anterior cranial fossa is formed by the frontal, ethmoid and sphenoid bones. It contains the frontal lobes of the brain. The greater part of the floor of the anterior cranial fossa consists of the frontal bone and it also forms the roof of the orbit. The part of the frontal bone that forms the anterior wall of the fossa contains the **frontal air sinus**. In the midline of the floor of the anterior cranial fossa is the ethmoid bone. In the midline a sharp ridge, the crista galli, provides attachment for the falx cerebri. In a depression on either side of the crista galli lie the **cribriform plates** of the ethmoid. These accommodate the **olfactory bulbs.** The bone of the cribriform plate is peppered with small perforations through which the fascicles of the olfactory nerve enter the cranial cavity from the nasal cavity to attach to the olfactory bulb.

Middle cranial fossa

The middle cranial fossa is formed by the sphenoid and temporal bones. In the midline, the body of the sphenoid forms a deep depression, the **hypophyseal fossa**, encompassed by four spurs of bone, the anterior and posterior clinoid processes. In the hypophyseal fossa lies the **hypophysis**, or **pituitary gland**. Lateral to the body of the sphenoid, the rest of the middle cranial fossa contains the temporal lobes of the cerebral hemisphere. The middle cranial fossa contains numerous points of entry and exit from the cranial cavity for cranial nerves and blood vessels. In particular:

- The **optic canal** is located medial to the anterior clinoid process and communicates with the orbit. Through it pass the optic (II) nerve and the ophthalmic artery (a branch of the internal carotid artery).
- The **superior orbital fissure** lies between the greater and lesser wings of the sphenoid bone and also communicates with the orbit. It carries the oculomotor (III), trochlear (IV) and abducens (VI) nerves and the ophthalmic division of the trigeminal (V) nerve.
- The **foramen rotundum** opens into the pterygopalatine fossa and carries the maxillary division of the trigeminal nerve.
- The **foramen ovale** carries the large mandibular division of the trigeminal nerve.
- The **foramen spinosum** is the point of entry of the middle meningeal artery.

 Raised intracranial pressure
A **space-occupying lesion** is an expanding focal lesion such as a tumour, haematoma or abscess. Since the cranial cavity is closed and unyielding, the brain is distorted and displaced downwards, towards the foramen magnum, as the intracranial pressure rises. The patient complains of headache, vomiting, blurring of vision and drowsiness. The optic discs are swollen (**papilloedema**), signs of brain stem dysfunction are found, and coma and death supervene if the pressure is not relieved by neurosurgery (craniotomy). **Benign intracranial hypertension** is caused by generalised swelling of the brain in the absence of a focal space-occupying lesion. It often occurs in obese young women; the syndrome of raised intracranial pressure mimics a brain tumour, hence the old designation, 'pseudo tumour cerebri'.

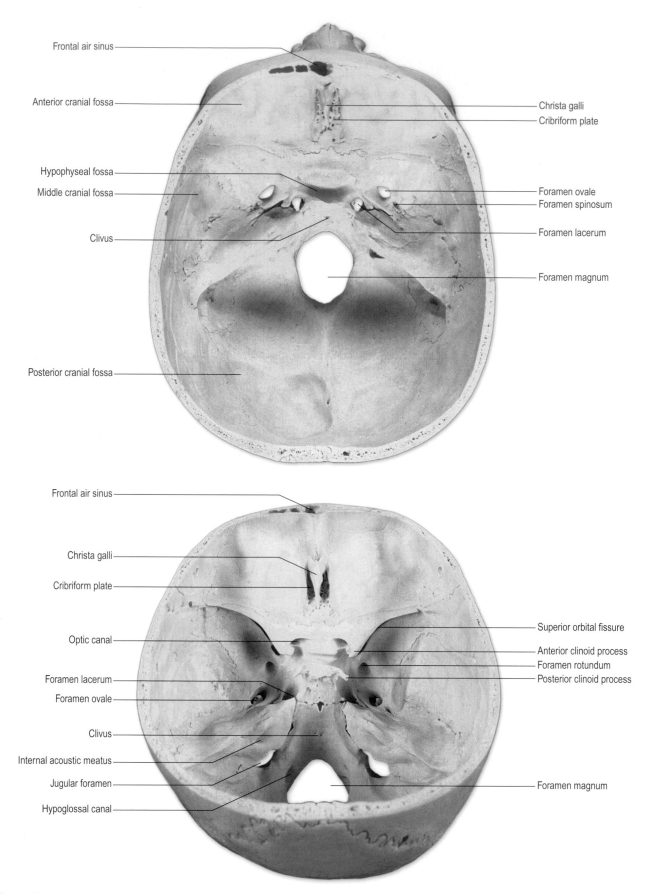

Figure 5.1 **Floor of the skull showing the three cranial fossae and principal foramina.**

Foraminal syndromes

The exit foramina of the skull represent sites of potential extrinsic compression of structures running through them, by disorders such as bony deformity and tumours of bone, meninges or blood vessels. The particular cranial nerves damaged at the exit site lead to 'foraminal syndromes', e.g. of the **superior orbital fissure** (see p. 102) or **jugular foramen** (see p. 110). The spinal cord, lower brain stem and the tonsils of the cerebellum are compromised in the **foramen magnum syndrome**.

Posterior cranial fossa

The posterior cranial fossa is formed by the occipital and petrous temporal bones. Anteriorly, in the midline, it forms a steep, smooth slope (the **clivus**) that is continuous with the body of the sphenoid bone, posterior to the hypophyseal fossa. The brain stem rests upon the clivus, the medulla passing through the **foramen magnum** to become continuous with the spinal cord. The foramen magnum also admits the vertebral arteries and the spinal root of the accessory (XI) nerve. In the lateral wall of the foramen magnum lies the **hypoglossal canal** through which the hypoglossal (XII) nerve leaves the cranial cavity. Between the occipital and petrous temporal bones lies the large **jugular foramen** through which pass the internal jugular vein, and the glossopharyngeal (IX), vagus (X) and accessory (XI) nerves. In the vertical wall of the petrous temporal bone is located the **internal auditory (acoustic) meatus**, which transmits the vestibulocochlear (VIII) and facial (VII) nerves. The cerebellum rests on the floor of the posterior cranial fossa.

Cranial meninges

Dura mater

The cranial dura is a tough, fibrous membrane that ensheathes the brain like a loose-fitting bag. In some regions, such as the floor of the cranial cavity and the midline of the cranial roof, the dura is tightly adherent to the interior surface of the skull, while elsewhere, such as the frontoparietal area, the two are separated by a narrow extradural space. Two large reflections of dura extend into the cranial cavity and occupy the fissures between major components of the brain (Figs 5.2, 5.3). In the midline, a vertical sheet of dura, the **falx cerebri**, extends from the cranial roof into the great longitudinal fissure between the cerebral hemispheres. The falx, therefore, has an attached border that adheres to the inner surface of the skull and a free border that lies above the corpus callosum. A horizontal shelf of dura, the **tentorium cerebelli**, extends inwards from the occipitotemporal region of the skull to lie in the transverse cerebral fissure, between the posterior part of the cerebral hemispheres and the cerebellum. The tentorium has a free border that encircles the midbrain, as the brain stem communicates between the posterior and middle cranial fossae. In the midline the tentorium becomes continuous superiorly with the falx cerebri.

Skull

- The bones of the skull and the meninges provide protection for the brain.
- The brain lies on the floor of the cranial cavity, which consists of three fossae.
- The anterior cranial fossa contains the frontal lobes of the cerebral hemispheres.
- It forms the roof of the orbit and is closely associated with the frontal air sinus.
- The cribriform plate admits the olfactory nerves to the cranial cavity and accommodates the olfactory bulb.
- The middle cranial fossa contains the temporal lobe. In the midline, the hypophyseal fossa holds the pituitary gland.
- A number of foramina provide entry and exit for important blood vessels and cranial nerves (indicated in parentheses):
  - Optic canal (optic nerve, ophthalmic artery)
  - Superior orbital fissure (oculomotor, trochlear, abducens and ophthalmic division of trigeminal nerves)
  - Foramen rotundum (maxillary division of trigeminal nerve)
  - Foramen ovale (mandibular division of trigeminal nerve)
  - Foramen spinosum (middle meningeal artery).
- The posterior cranial fossa accommodates the brain stem and cerebellum.
- A number of important structures pass through the foramina of the posterior fossa:
  - *Foramen magnum* (medulla oblongata, vertebral arteries, spinal root of the accessory nerve)
  - *Hypoglossal canal* (hypoglossal nerve)
  - *Jugular foramen* (internal jugular vein, glossopharyngeal, vagus and accessory nerves)
  - *Internal auditory meatus* (facial and vestibulocochlear nerves).

Head trauma

Head trauma, especially resulting from road traffic accidents, is the most common cause of death and disability in youth. The injury may be blunt ('closed') or caused by a penetrating missile. The skull may be fractured and depressed, tearing brain coverings and the brain itself. Displacement and torsion of the brain lead to contusion, tearing of white matter and bleeding into the brain (**intracerebral haematoma**), causing unconsciousness (concussion), neurological and psychological deficits, and post-traumatic epilepsy.

Tearing of the middle meningeal artery causes bleeding into the extradural space (**extradural haematoma**). As the blood clot expands, the brain is compressed; as a result, coma supervenes a delayed period of hours after the blow. Without neurosurgical evacuation, the rising intracranial pressure causes brain displacement and death.

Tearing of the veins stretching across the subdural space causes gradual seepage of blood, collecting to form a chronic **subdural haematoma** with eventual coma. The delay between the blow and the development of symptoms may be of weeks or months. The elderly are particularly vulnerable and the head injury may be slight and forgotten. Again, surgical removal of the clot is life-saving.

Falx cerebri

Optic chiasma

Midbrain

Tentorium cerebelli

Figure 5.2 **Cranial cavity showing the arrangement of the dura mater.**

Corpus callosum

Cerebral hemisphere

Interpeduncular cistern

Pituitary gland

Pons

Medulla

Falx cerebri

Thalamus

Midbrain

Tentorium cerebelli

Cerebellum

Cisterna magna

Figure 5.3 **Paramedian sagittal section of the head, showing the disposition of the brain and meninges.**

Arachnoid mater and pia mater

The arachnoid mater is a soft, translucent membrane that, like the dura mater, loosely envelops the brain (Figs 1.13, 6.10). It is separated from the dura by a narrow subdural space, through which pass veins en route to the dural venous sinuses (Ch. 7).

The pia mater is a microscopically thin, delicate and highly vascular membrane that is closely adherent to the surface of the brain, following all its concavities and convexities. Between the pia and arachnoid mater lies the **subarachnoid space**. This contains a filamentous network of connective tissue strands (trabeculae) and is traversed by numerous arteries and veins. It also contains CSF, which is produced by the choroid plexus within the cerebral ventricles (Ch. 6). Since the arachnoid mater fits loosely round the brain while the pia closely follows its surface contours, the subarachnoid space is of greatly varying depth in different regions. Where significant depressions or fissures in the brain are spanned by the arachnoid mater, **subarachnoid cisterns** are formed. Two of these are particularly large:

- The **cisterna magna** lies between the cerebellum and the dorsal surface of the medulla (Figs 5.3, 5.4). Into this cistern flows CSF from the fourth ventricle.
- The **interpeduncular cistern** is located at the base of the brain (Fig. 5.3), where the arachnoid spans the space between the two temporal lobes. This cistern contains the optic chiasma. The cistern is deepest between the two cerebral peduncles of the midbrain.

Dural venous sinuses

The dura mater is considered to be comprised of two layers. These are normally closely adherent to one another but, in certain locations, become separated to enclose blood-filled spaces, the dural venous sinuses. Major venous sinuses lie in the attached borders of the falx cerebri and tentorium cerebelli and also on the floor of the cranial cavity. Venous blood from the brain flows into the sinuses through a series of venous channels and in turn the sinuses drain principally into the internal jugular vein, through which blood is returned to the general extracranial circulation. The dural venous sinuses are described further in Chapter 7, which deals with the blood supply to the CNS.

Cerebellar hemisphere

Arachnoid mater covering cisterna magna

Medulla

Figure 5.4 **Cisterna magna.**

Cranial meninges

- The dura mater is the outermost meningeal membrane. Two dural sheets or reflections extend into the cranial cavity:
  - The falx cerebri, lying between the two cerebral hemispheres
  - The tentorium cerebelli, lying between the cerebellum and the occipital lobes of the cerebrum and encircling the midbrain.
- The dura contains a number of venous sinuses, which are important in the venous drainage of the brain.
- Important sinuses lie within the falx cerebri, tentorium cerebelli and on the floor of the cranial cavity.
- The middle meningeal layer is the arachnoid mater. Both the dura and arachnoid surround the brain loosely.
- The innermost meningeal layer is the pia mater, which adheres to the surface of the brain, closely following its contours. This creates a subarachnoid space of variable depth.
- The subarachnoid space contains CSF, which is secreted by the choroid plexus within the cerebral ventricles.

Meningitis

Inflammation of the meninges may result from infection with viruses (e.g. lymphocytic choriomeningitis), bacteria (meningococcal and tuberculous meningitis) or other organisms, or from chemical reaction to injected contrast medium during neuroradiological procedures. The patient complains of headache, photophobia and vomiting, is febrile and has neck stiffness on attempting to move the head. Viral and chemical meningitis are normally mild and self-limiting. Bacterial or fungal meningitis, however, leads to damage to cranial nerves and the brain itself; if untreated, it proceeds to raised intracranial pressure, brain displacement and death.

Chapter 6
Ventricular system and cerebrospinal fluid

The CNS contains an interconnecting series of chambers and channels that are derived from the lumen of the embryonic neural tube. In the spinal cord, this is represented by the vestigial and insignificant central canal. Within the brain, however, the enormous growth and distortion of the original tube-like structure is paralleled by the development of an elaborate system of ventricles (Figs 1.18, 6.1, 6.2).

Topographical anatomy of the ventricular system

In passing from the spinal cord to the brain stem, the central canal moves progressively more dorsal until, in the rostral (open) medulla, it opens out into a wide and shallow depression, the **fourth ventricle** (Fig. 6.3), which lies on the dorsal surface of the brain stem beneath the cerebellum. The fourth ventricle is rhomboid or diamond-shaped. On each side, a **lateral recess** extends towards the lateral margin of the brain stem and is in continuity, through a small **lateral aperture** (the **foramen of Luschka**), with the subarachnoid space of the cerebellopontine angle (Fig. 6.4). For the most part, the roof of the fourth ventricle is formed by the cerebellum. However, the roof of the caudal part consists of pia and ependyma, a central defect in which constitutes the **median aperture** of the fourth ventricle, or the **foramen of Magendie**, that provides communication with the cisterna magna (Fig. 6.5). The rostral part of the roof of the fourth ventricle is partly formed by the superior cerebellar peduncles on either side, the space between them being bridged by the thin superior medullary velum.

The fourth ventricle extends rostrally as far as the pontomesencephalic junction where it becomes continuous with the **cerebral aqueduct**, which passes throughout the length of the midbrain, beneath the inferior and superior colliculi. At the rostral margin of the midbrain, the cerebral aqueduct opens into the **third ventricle**, which is a narrow slit-like cavity whose lateral walls are formed by the thalamus and hypothalamus on either side (Fig. 6.2 and see Fig. 12.2). The roof of the ventricle is formed by pia-ependyma, which spans between two nerve fibre bundles, the **striae medullaris thalami**, which are situated along the dorsomedial border of the thalamus. In the rostral part of the third ventricle lies an aperture, the **interventricular foramen** or **foramen of Monro**, which is located between the column of the fornix and the anterior pole of the thalamus.

The interventricular foramen provides communication, on either side, with the extensive **lateral ventricle** located within the cerebral hemisphere (Fig. 6.6 and see Fig. 16.12). The lateral ventricle is approximately C-shaped. It consists of an anterior (frontal) horn, body, posterior (occipital) horn and inferior (temporal) horn. The anterior horn of the lateral ventricle is that part anterior to the interventricular foramen. Its lateral wall is the head of the caudate nucleus and its roof is the corpus callosum (see Figs 13.3–13.7). The medial wall is formed by the **septum pellucidum**. This thin sheet spans between the corpus callosum and fornix in the midline and separates the anterior horns of the two lateral ventricles. The body of the lateral ventricle extends behind the interventricular foramen, having as its floor the thalamus and tail of the caudate nucleus. More posteriorly, the small posterior horn extends towards the occipital pole but the principal course of the ventricle sweeps downwards and forwards to form the extensive inferior horn, which lies in the temporal lobe. In the floor of the inferior horn lies the hippocampus, while in its roof runs the much attenuated tail of the caudate nucleus (see Figs 13.9–13.12 and 16.12).

> ## Topographical anatomy
>
> - The ventricular system consists of the lateral ventricles, third ventricle, cerebral aqueduct and fourth ventricle.
> - The lateral ventricle is located within each cerebral hemisphere and is approximately C-shaped. It communicates, via the interventricular foramen, with the third ventricle.
> - The third ventricle is a midline, slit-like cavity. Its lateral walls consist of the thalamus and hypothalamus. Caudally, the third ventricle becomes continuous with the cerebral aqueduct.
> - The cerebral aqueduct extends throughout the midbrain, linking the third and fourth ventricles.
> - The fourth ventricle is located between the brain stem (pons and medulla) and the cerebellum. A median aperture and two lateral apertures communicate with the subarachnoid space surrounding the brain.

Cerebrospinal fluid

The ventricular system, together with the cranial and spinal subarachnoid spaces, contains cerebrospinal fluid (CSF; Fig. 6.7). This is produced by the **choroid plexus**, which is located in the lateral, third and fourth ventricles (Figs 6.2, 6.6 and see Fig. 16.12). The choroid plexus is formed by invagination of the vascular pia mater into the ventricular

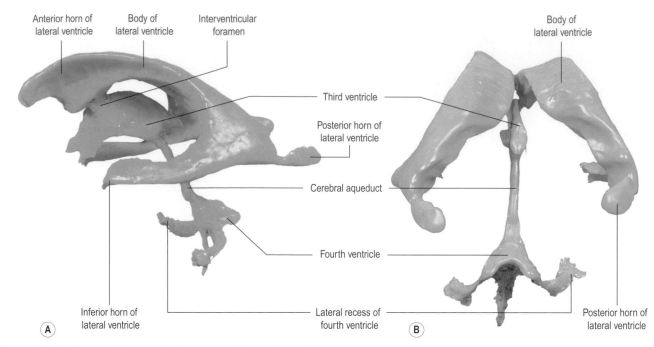

Anterior horn of lateral ventricle

Body of lateral ventricle

Interventricular foramen

Body of lateral ventricle

Third ventricle

Posterior horn of lateral ventricle

Cerebral aqueduct

Fourth ventricle

Inferior horn of lateral ventricle

Lateral recess of fourth ventricle

Posterior horn of lateral ventricle

(A)

(B)

Figure 6.1 **Resin cast of the ventricular system. (A)** Lateral view; **(B)** posterior view.

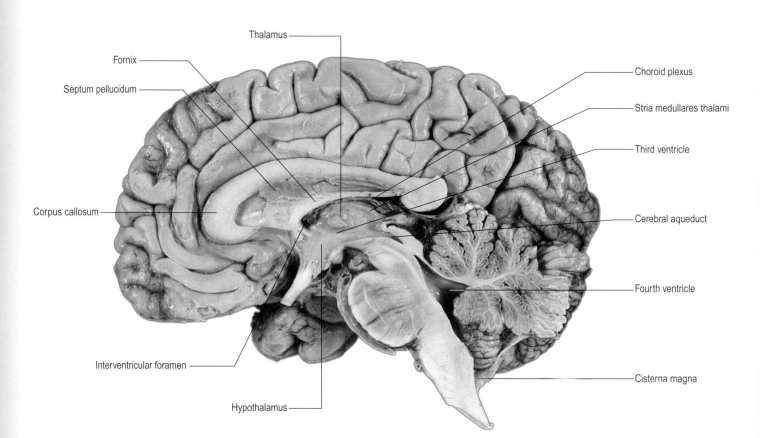

Thalamus

Fornix

Septum pellucidum

Choroid plexus

Stria medullares thalami

Third ventricle

Corpus callosum

Cerebral aqueduct

Fourth ventricle

Interventricular foramen

Cisterna magna

Hypothalamus

Figure 6.2 **Median sagittal section of the brain showing the ventricular system.**

Superior cerebellar peduncle

Inferior colliculus of midbrain

Middle cerebellar peduncle

Floor of fourth ventricle

Inferior cerebellar peduncle

Lateral recess and aperture of fourth venticle

Medulla oblongata

Figure 6.3 **Dorsal aspect of brain stem illustrating the floor of the fourth ventricle.**

Pons   Basilar artery   Choroid plexus   Facial nerve

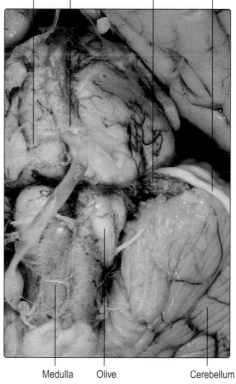

Medulla   Olive   Cerebellum

Figure 6.4 **Cerebellopontine angle.** The point of continuity between the lateral recess of the fourth ventricle and the subarachnoid space is indicated by a small tuft of choroid plexus, which protrudes through the lateral aperture.

Superior vermis of cerebellum

Median aperture of fourth ventricle

Dorsal aspect of medulla   Cerebellar hemisphere

Figure 6.5 **Posterior view of the brain.** The cerebellum and brain stem have been slightly separated to show the median aperture of the fourth ventricle.

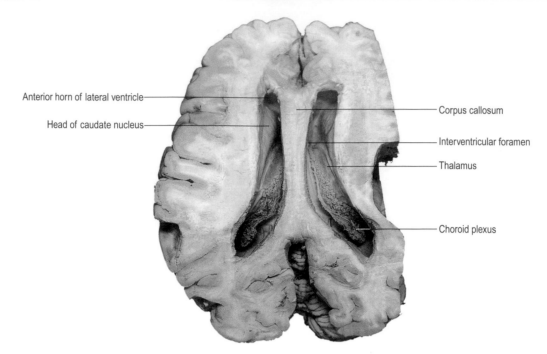

Figure 6.6 **Superior aspect of a dissection of the cerebral hemispheres in which much of the corpus callosum has been removed to reveal the lumen of the lateral ventricles.**

Figure 6.7 **Sagittal T$_2$-weighted MR image of the brain demonstrating CSF within the ventricular system and subarachnoid space.** (Courtesy of Professor A Jackson, Wolfson Molecular Imaging Centre, University of Manchester, Manchester, UK.)

lumen, where it becomes highly convoluted, producing a sponge-like appearance. The choroid plexus enters the third and fourth ventricles through their roofs and the lateral ventricle through the choroid fissure, along the line of the fimbria/fornix (see Figs 16.8, 16.12).

CSF is produced partly by an active secretory process and partly by passive diffusion. It is a colourless fluid containing little protein and few cells. The volume of CSF in the combined ventricular and subarachnoid spaces is approximately 150 mL. CSF is produced continuously, at a rate sufficient to fill these spaces several times each day. This means that an efficient mechanism is required for the circulation of CSF and its reabsorption (Figs 6.8–6.10).

Most CSF is produced by the choroid plexus of the lateral ventricle. From here it flows through the interventricular foramen into the third ventricle and thence, by way of the cerebral aqueduct, into the fourth ventricle. CSF leaves the ventricular system through the three apertures of the fourth ventricle and, thus, enters the subarachnoid space. Most CSF passes through the median aperture to enter the cisterna magna, located between the medulla and cerebellum. A lesser amount flows through the lateral apertures to enter the subarachnoid space in the region of the cerebellopontine angle. From these sites, the majority of CSF flows superiorly, round the cerebral hemispheres, to the sites of reabsorption. Within the subarachnoid space, CSF

Figure 6.8 **The cerebral ventricular system and its relationship with the subarachnoid space.** The circulation of cerebrospinal fluid is indicated by arrows.

Figure 6.9 **Transverse section through the superior sagittal sinus showing arachnoid villi.**

Figure 6.10 **Superior aspect of the cerebral hemispheres showing arachnoid granulations on the right side.** On the left side, the arachnoid mater has been removed.

serves partially to cushion the brain from sudden movements of the head.

CSF is reabsorbed into the venous system by passing into the dural venous sinuses, principally the superior sagittal sinus. Along the sinuses are located numerous **arachnoid villi**, which consist of invaginations of arachnoid mater through the dural wall and into the lumen of the sinus

(Fig. 6.9). Reabsorption occurs at these sites because the hydrostatic pressure in the subarachnoid space is higher than that in the lumen of the sinus and because of the greater colloid osmotic pressure of venous blood compared to CSF. With age, the arachnoid villi become hypertrophic to form **arachnoid granulations** (Fig. 6.10)

Hydrocephalus

Obstruction of the flow of CSF within the ventricular system (e.g. by tumours) or the subarachnoid space (e.g. by adhesions following head injury or meningitis) leads to a rise in fluid pressure causing swelling of the ventricles (**hydrocephalus**). The clinical effects are similar to those of a brain tumour and consist of headaches, unsteadiness and mental impairment. Swelling of the optic discs (**papilloedema**) is seen on ophthalmoscopy. Decompression of the dilated ventricles is achieved by inserting a shunt connecting the ventricles to the jugular vein or the abdominal peritoneum.

Cerebrospinal fluid

- Each ventricle contains choroid plexus, which secretes CSF.
- CSF flows in the direction: lateral ventricle → third ventricle → cerebral aqueduct → fourth ventricle → subarachnoid space.
- The combined ventricular system and subarachnoid space contains about 150 mL CSF, this volume being produced several times each day.
- CSF is reabsorbed into the venous system through arachnoid villi, which project principally into the superior sagittal sinus.

Chapter 7
Blood supply of the central nervous system

Blood supply of the spinal cord

Arterial supply of the spinal cord

Three longitudinal arterial vessels run the length of the spinal cord (Fig. 7.1). These are the single **anterior spinal artery** and the paired **posterior spinal arteries**. The anterior spinal artery arises in a Y-shaped configuration from the two vertebral arteries at the level of the medulla (Fig. 7.2) and descends along the ventral surface of the cord in the midline. The posterior spinal arteries arise from either the vertebral arteries or the posterior inferior cerebellar arteries and run caudally on the posterolateral surface of the cord.

The anterior and posterior spinal arteries alone are insufficient to supply the cord below cervical levels and, therefore, they receive serial reinforcement by anastomosis with **radicular arteries** derived from segmental vessels, including the ascending cervical, intercostal and lumbar arteries. Radicular arteries pass through the intervertebral foramina and divide into anterior and posterior branches, which run with the dorsal and ventral spinal nerve roots, respectively. One particularly large radicular artery (the **great radicular artery**, or **artery of Adamkiewicz**) may arise from a lateral intercostal or lumbar artery at any level from T8–L3.

Disorders of blood supply of the spinal cord

The blood supply of the spinal cord is most vulnerable in the thoracic region and in the anterior portion of the cord. **Occlusion of the anterior spinal artery** leads to an acute thoracic cord syndrome with paraplegia and incontinence. The spinothalamic modalities of pain and temperature are preferentially lost, whereas the proprioceptive functions of the dorsal columns are relatively preserved.

Venous drainage of the spinal cord

The venous drainage of the cord follows a basically similar pattern to the arterial supply (Fig. 7.1). Six longitudinal interconnecting venous channels exist. These consist primarily of **anterior** and **posterior spinal veins**, which run in the midline. More irregular, sometimes incomplete, bilaterally paired **anterolateral** and **posterolateral veins** are situated near the lines of attachment of the ventral and dorsal nerve roots, respectively. All of these vessels drain via **anterior** and **posterior radicular veins** into the **internal vertebral venous plexus** (epidural venous plexus), which is situated between the dura mater and the vertebral periosteum. The internal venous plexus communicates with an **external vertebral venous plexus** and thence with the ascending lumbar veins, the azygos and hemiazygos veins.

Blood supply of the spinal cord

- The spinal cord is supplied by the anterior and posterior spinal arteries, supplemented by radicular arteries.
- Venous drainage is by anterior and posterior spinal veins which drain, via radicular veins, into the internal vertebral venous plexus.

Blood supply of the brain

Arterial supply of the brain

The brain is supplied with blood by two pairs of vessels, the internal carotid arteries and the vertebral arteries (Figs 7.2, 7.3 and see Fig. 7.7). The **internal carotid artery** arises from the common carotid artery and enters the middle fossa of the cranial cavity through the carotid canal. Its course then follows a series of characteristic bends, known as the **carotid syphon** (Fig. 7.4), after which it passes forwards through the cavernous sinus and then upwards on the medial aspect of the anterior clinoid process, reaching the surface of the brain lateral to the optic chiasma. Along its course, the internal carotid artery gives rise to a number of preterminal branches.

- **Hypophyseal arteries** arise from the intracavernous section of the internal carotid to supply the neurohypophysis. They also form the pituitary portal system of vessels by which releasing factors are carried from the hypothalamus to the adenohypophysis (Ch. 16).
- The **ophthalmic artery** passes into the orbit through the optic foramen. It supplies the structures of the orbit, the frontal and ethmoidal sinuses, the frontal part of the scalp and dorsum of the nose.
- The **anterior choroidal artery** supplies the optic tract, the choroid plexus of the lateral ventricle, the hippocampus and some of the deep structures of the

Figure 7.1 **The arterial supply and venous drainage of the spinal cord.**

Figure 7.2 **The arrangement of arterial vessels on the base of the brain.** The diagram shows the circulus arteriosus (circle of Willis).

Anterior cerebral artery

Optic nerve

Cut end of internal carotid artery

Posterior communicating artery

Pontine arteries

Posterior inferior cerebellar artery

Hypoglossal nerve roots

Middle cerebral artery

Oculomotor nerve

Posterior cerebral artery

Superior cerebellar artery

Basilar artery

Trigeminal nerve

Anterior inferior cerebellar artery

Vertebral artery

Anterior spinal artery

Figure 7.3 **Arteries on the base of the brain.** The arterial system has been injected with a red resin.

hemisphere, including the internal capsule and globus pallidus.

■ The **posterior communicating artery** passes backwards to join the posterior cerebral artery, thus forming part of the circle of Willis.

Lateral to the optic chiasma, the internal carotid artery divides into its two terminal branches, the **anterior** and **middle cerebral arteries**. The anterior cerebral artery courses medially above the optic nerve and then passes into the great longitudinal fissure, between the frontal lobes of the cerebral hemispheres. As it does so, it is joined to the corresponding vessel of the opposite side by the short **anterior communicating artery**. Within the great longitudinal fissure, the anterior cerebral artery follows the dorsal curvature of the corpus callosum (Fig. 13.24), branches ramifying over the medial surface of the frontal and parietal lobes, which it supplies (Fig. 7.5). The territory

supplied by the anterior cerebral artery, therefore, includes the motor and sensory cortices for the lower limb. Fine terminal branches also extend out of the great longitudinal fissure to supply a narrow lateral band of frontal and parietal cortices.

The middle cerebral artery is the largest of the three cerebral arteries and its cortical territory is the most extensive (Fig. 7.5). It passes laterally from its origin to enter the lateral fissure within which it subdivides, its branches supplying virtually the whole of the lateral surface of the frontal, parietal and temporal lobes. This territory includes the primary motor and sensory cortices for the whole of the body, excluding the lower limb. It also serves the auditory cortex and the insula within the depths of the lateral fissure.

Since the structures supplied by branches of the internal carotid artery are normally perfused almost entirely from this source, they are often referred to as being supplied by the 'internal carotid system'.

Figure 7.4 **Carotid angiograms.** Radio-opaque material has been introduced into the internal carotid artery in order to display its intracranial course and the distribution of its branches. **(A)** Left carotid, lateral view; **(B)** Right carotid, frontal view. (Courtesy of Professor P D Griffiths, Academic Unit of Radiology, University of Sheffield, Sheffield, UK.)

Figure 7.5 **The cerebral cortical distribution of the anterior, middle and posterior cerebral arteries. (A)** Lateral aspect; **(B)** Medial aspect.

The **vertebral artery** arises from the subclavian artery, ascends through the foramina transversaria of the cervical vertebrae and enters the cranial cavity through the foramen magnum, alongside the ventrolateral aspect of the medulla (Figs 7.2, 7.3, 7.6, 7.7). As they pass rostrally, the two vertebral arteries converge, uniting at the junction of the medulla and pons to form the midline **basilar artery**. Along its course, the vertebral artery gives rise to a number of branches, including the anterior and posterior spinal arteries, which supply the medulla and spinal cord. Its largest branch is the **posterior inferior cerebellar artery**, which supplies the inferior aspect of the cerebellum.

The basilar artery runs the length of the pons, which it supplies by means of many small **pontine branches**. It also gives rise to the **anterior inferior cerebellar artery**, which supplies the anterior and inferior portion of the cerebellum, and the **labyrinthine artery**, which passes into the internal acoustic meatus to supply the inner ear. At the junction of the pons and midbrain, the basilar artery divides into two pairs of vessels, the **superior cerebellar arteries** and the **posterior cerebral arteries**. The superior cerebellar artery supplies the superior aspect of the cerebellum. The posterior cerebral artery curves around the midbrain to supply the visual cortex of the occipital lobe and the inferomedial aspect of the temporal lobe (Fig. 7.5).

The brain regions (brain stem, cerebellum and occipital lobe) served by the vertebral and basilar arteries and their branches are described as being supplied by the 'vertebrobasilar system'.

The internal carotid and vertebrobasilar systems are joined by two thin vessels, the **posterior communicating arteries**, which pass rostrocaudally between the ends of the internal carotid arteries and the posterior cerebral arteries.

This completes an anastomosis of vessels on the base of the brain, known as the **circulus arteriosus** or **circle of Willis** (Figs 7.2, 7.3), which encircles the optic chiasma and the floor of the hypothalamus and midbrain. The anastomotic arrangement of vessels provides the possibility that obstruction or narrowing of the proximal parts of the

Figure 7.6 **Vertebral angiograms.** Radio-opaque material has been introduced into the vertebral artery in order to display its intracranial course and the distribution of its branches. **(A)** Lateral view; **(B)** Frontal view. (Courtesy of Professor P D Griffiths, Academic Unit of Radiology, University of Sheffield, Sheffield, UK.)

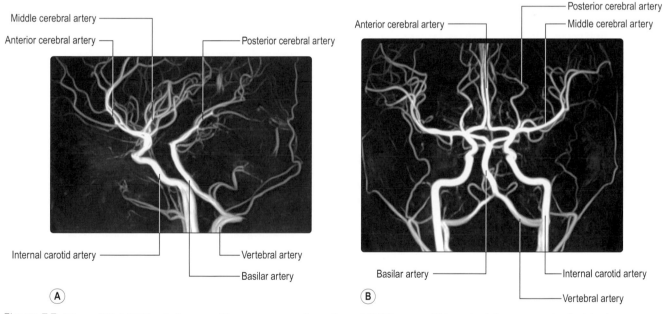

Figure 7.7 **'Time-of-flight' MR arteriograms.** The scans were performed on a 3.0T MR scanner. This method does not require the injection of contrast media into the patient; rather it relies on complex MR sequences to produce signal from structures with flow, while suppressing signal from stationary tissues. **(A)** Lateral view; **(B)** Frontal view. (Courtesy of Professor P D Griffiths, Academic Unit of Radiology, University of Sheffield, Sheffield, UK.)

cerebral arteries, which would be expected to lead to insufficiency in the perfusion of their territories, might be compensated by circulation of blood through the communicating arteries. The actual significance of this arrangement is dependent upon the size of the communicating arteries, which is highly variable between individuals. From the arteries that constitute the circle of Willis, numerous small vessels penetrate the surface of the brain. These are known as **perforating arteries** (central or ganglionic arteries) and consist of two main groups:

1. **Anterior perforating arteries,** which arise from the anterior cerebral artery, anterior communicating artery and the region of origin of the middle cerebral artery. They enter the brain in the region between the optic chiasma and the termination of the olfactory tract, known as the **anterior perforated substance** (Fig. 16.13). These vessels supply large parts of the basal ganglia, the optic chiasma, the internal capsule and the hypothalamus.

2. **Posterior perforating arteries,** which arise from the posterior cerebral and posterior communicating arteries. They enter the brain in the region between the two crura cerebri of the midbrain, known as the **posterior perforated substance** (Fig. 16.13), to supply the ventral portion of the midbrain and parts of the subthalamus and hypothalamus.

Disorders of blood supply of the brain

One of the most common causes of neurological disability is **stroke**. The sudden occlusion of a cerebral artery leads to death of brain tissue (**infarction**). Rupture of a blood vessel causes bleeding into the brain (**cerebral haemorrhage**). These events lead to the rapid development of a focal neurological syndrome. Strokes related to the carotid artery and its cerebral branches are associated with focal epilepsy, a contralateral sensory/motor deficit and a psychological deficit (e.g. aphasia). Strokes involving the vertebrobasilar circulation lead to a focal brain stem syndrome. Recovery of function can occur but may take up to 2 years and can be incomplete.

An **aneurysm** is an abnormal, balloon-like, swelling of an artery. A surgical emergency arises when an aneurysm ruptures and blood projects around the brain in the subarachnoid space (**subarachnoid haemorrhage**) and into the brain (**intracerebral haemorrhage**). A sudden severe headache and neck stiffness are followed by coma and neurological deficits. Neurosurgery or intra-arterial 'coiling' are required to seal the aneurysm to prevent further bleeding and allow recovery.

An **angioma**, or **arteriovenous malformation**, is a congenital collection of swollen blood vessels that can rupture, causing cerebral haemorrhage, or 'steal' blood from adjacent brain regions, leading to epilepsy and a focal cerebral syndrome.

Arterial supply of the brain

- The brain is supplied by paired internal carotid and vertebral arteries.
- The internal carotid artery terminates lateral to the optic chiasma, giving rise to the anterior and middle cerebral arteries.
- The anterior cerebral artery passes into the great longitudinal fissure and supplies the medial aspect of the cerebral hemisphere.
- The middle cerebral artery passes into the lateral fissure and supplies the lateral aspect of the cerebral hemisphere.
- The vertebral arteries run on the ventrolateral aspect of the medulla, uniting to form the midline basilar artery, which extends the length of the pons. Along their course the vertebral and basilar arteries give rise to branches that supply the cerebellum and brain stem.
- The principal terminal branch of the basilar artery is the posterior cerebral artery, which supplies the occipital lobe of the cerebral hemisphere.
- The anterior communicating artery links together the two anterior cerebral arteries. Posterior communicating arteries pass between the internal carotid artery and the posterior cerebral artery, on each side. This anastomosis of vessels constitutes the circle of Willis.
- Small perforating arteries arise from the circle of Willis to supply the hypothalamic area, the basal ganglia and the internal capsule.

Venous drainage of the brain

Three sorts of vessels contribute to the venous drainage of the brain (Figs 7.8–7.10): deep veins, superficial veins and the dural venous sinuses. None of these vessels contains valves.

Deep cerebral veins drain the internal structures of the forebrain (Fig. 7.8). Of particular note are the **thalamostriate vein** and the **choroidal vein**, which drain the basal ganglia, thalamus, internal capsule, choroid plexus and hippocampus. Within each cerebral hemisphere, these vessels merge to form the **internal cerebral vein**. The two internal cerebral veins then unite in the midline to form the **great cerebral vein** (of Galen), which lies beneath the splenium of the corpus callosum. This short vessel is continuous with the straight sinus, which lies in the midline of the tentorium cerebelli.

Superficial veins lie within the subarachnoid space (Fig. 7.9). **Superior cerebral veins** primarily drain the lateral surface of the cerebral hemispheres and empty into the superior sagittal sinus. The **superficial middle cerebral vein** runs along the line of the lateral fissure and empties into the cavernous sinus. In addition, two major anastomotic channels exist, the superior (great) anastomotic vein and the inferior anastomotic vein, which drain into the superior sagittal sinus and the transverse sinus, respectively.

The deep and superficial cerebral veins drain into the **dural venous sinuses** (Figs 7.9, 7.10; see also Ch. 5), which are channels formed between the two layers of dura mater. Major venous sinuses are located in the attached borders of the falx cerebri and the tentorium cerebelli, and on the floor of the cranial cavity.

Along the line where the falx cerebri attaches to the interior of the cranium lies the **superior sagittal sinus**. This receives blood primarily from the superior cerebral veins, which ramify over the lateral surface of the cerebral hemispheres. The free border of the falx encloses the smaller **inferior sagittal sinus**, into which flow veins on the medial aspect of the hemisphere. Within the tentorium cerebelli, along the line of its attachment to the falx, lies the large **straight sinus**. Into this run both the great cerebral vein, which drains the deep structures of the forebrain, and the inferior sagittal sinus.

The superior sagittal sinus and the straight sinus converge at the **confluence of the sinuses**, which lies adjacent to the internal occipital protuberance. From here, blood flows laterally on either side in the **transverse sinus**, which lies along the line of attachment of the tentorium to the occipital bone. The transverse sinus is continuous with the **sigmoid sinus**, which, in turn, joins the **internal jugular vein** at the level of the jugular foramen.

The **cavernous sinus** (Fig. 7.11) lies lateral to the body of the sphenoid bone. It receives blood from the middle cerebral vein and drains into the internal jugular vein (via the inferior petrosal sinus) and into the transverse sinus (via the superior petrosal sinus). The two cavernous sinuses are connected by intercavernous sinuses that lie anterior and posterior to the hypophysis, forming a venous circle around it (the circular sinus). The dural venous sinuses are connected to extracranial veins via **emissary veins**.

Figure 7.8 **The deep cerebral veins.** The brain is viewed from above and the corpus callosum has been removed to reveal the third and lateral ventricles.

Figure 7.9 **Venous drainage of the brain. (A)** Lateral view; **(B)** Sagittal view.

Diseases of the venous sinuses

Thrombosis of the sagittal sinuses is a rare complication of childbirth, blood-clotting disorders and ear infection. Obstruction of the venous drainage of the brain leads to cerebral swelling (**oedema**) and the syndrome of **raised intracranial pressure** (see p. 47). Cerebral damage caused by venous infarction manifests as epileptic seizures and focal paralysis of the limbs.

In **cavernous sinus thrombosis** there is acute pain and swelling of the orbit and contents, with ophthalmoplegia, ptosis and numbness of the face.

Superior sagittal sinus

Cortical veins

Transverse sinus

Superior sagittal sinus

(A)

Sigmoid sinus

Great cerebral vein

Straight sinus

Transverse sinus

Confluence of sinuses

(B)

Confluence of sinuses

Sigmoid sinus

Figure 7.10 **Phase contrast MR venograms.** The scans were performed on a 3.0T MR scanner. **(A)** Lateral view; **(B)** Frontal view. (Courtesy of Professor P D Griffiths, Academic Unit of Radiology, University of Sheffield, Sheffield, UK.)

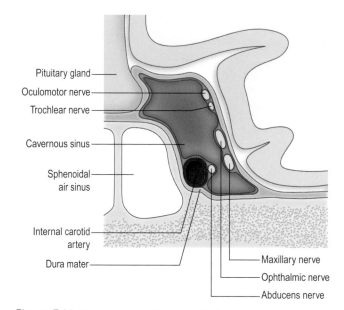

Pituitary gland

Oculomotor nerve

Trochlear nerve

Cavernous sinus

Sphenoidal air sinus

Internal carotid artery

Dura mater

Maxillary nerve

Ophthalmic nerve

Abducens nerve

Figure 7.11 **Transverse section through the cavernous sinus.**

Venous drainage of the brain

- Venous drainage of the brain involves deep veins, superficial veins and dural venous sinuses.
- Deep cerebral veins drain into the great cerebral vein, which is continuous with the straight sinus.
- Superficial veins empty principally into the superior sagittal sinus and the cavernous sinus.
- The superior sagittal sinus and straight sinuses meet at the confluence of the sinuses.
- Venous blood flows, via the transverse sinus and sigmoid sinus, into the internal jugular vein.

Chapter 8
Spinal cord

The spinal cord and its associated spinal nerves are of immense functional importance. These structures act to:

- receive afferent fibres from sensory receptors of the trunk and limbs
- control movements of the trunk and limbs
- provide autonomic innervation for most of the viscera.

The internal organisation of the cord permits many functions to operate in an automatic or reflex fashion. In addition, extensive connections with the brain, through ascending and descending nerve fibre tracts, both convey afferent information to higher centres and mediate their controlling influence over spinal mechanisms.

External features of the spinal cord

Topographical anatomy
The spinal cord occupies the vertebral (or spinal) canal within the vertebral column, which provides support and protection (Figs 8.1, 8.2). Rostrally, the cord is continuous with the medulla oblongata of the brain stem.

The spinal cord is essentially a segmental structure; from rostral to caudal, it consists of 8 cervical (C), 12 thoracic (T), 5 lumbar (L), 5 sacral (S) and 1 coccygeal segments (Fig. 8.3). The cord is approximately cylindrical in shape but its diameter varies considerably at different levels. It bears two enlargements, cervical and lumbar. The **cervical enlargement** consists of cord segments C4–T1 and provides innervation for the upper limb via the **brachial plexus** (see Fig. 3.11). The **lumbar enlargement** is made up of segments L1–S3 and is associated with innervation of the lower limb via the **lumbosacral plexus** (see Fig. 3.13). Caudal to the lumbar enlargement, the cord tapers abruptly to form a conical termination, the **conus medullaris**. From the tip of the conus, a strand of connective tissue, the **filum terminale** (Fig. 8.4), extends caudally and is attached to the dorsal surface of the first coccygeal vertebra.

Until the third month of fetal life, the spinal cord occupies the entire length of the vertebral canal. Thereafter, the rate of elongation of the vertebral column exceeds that of the spinal cord; as a result, at birth the cord terminates at the level of the third lumbar vertebra (L3) and in adult life, it terminates at the level of the intervertebral disc between L1 and L2 (Figs 8.3, 8.4).

The approximate location of spinal cord segments relative to the bony vertebrae may be identified in the living subject by reference to the posterior spinous processes of the vertebrae. As a rule-of-thumb, cervical cord segments lie approximately one spine higher than their corresponding vertebrae (e.g. C7 cord segment lies adjacent to C6 vertebra), thoracic segments lie approximately two spines higher, and lumbar segments three to four spines higher than their corresponding vertebrae (Fig. 8.3).

> ## Topographical anatomy
>
> - The spinal cord provides sensory, motor and autonomic innervation for the trunk and limbs.
> - The cord possesses two enlargements: cervical (C4–T1), associated with innervation of the upper limbs, and lumbar (L1–S3), innervating the lower limbs.
> - The cord terminates at vertebral level L1–L2 in the adult.

Spinal nerves
The spinal cord bears 31 bilaterally paired spinal nerves, each pair being associated with its corresponding cord segment. The spinal nerves originate as two linear series of nerve fascicles, or rootlets, attached to the dorsolateral and ventrolateral aspects of the cord (Fig. 8.5). The groups of six to eight contiguous fascicles that are attached to each cord segment coalesce to form **dorsal** and **ventral nerve roots**. The dorsal and ventral roots of each cord segment then pass to their corresponding **intervertebral foramen** (Fig. 8.6), in or near which they join to form the spinal nerve proper. While the spinal nerves are mixed nerves, containing both afferent and efferent neurones, the dorsal and ventral roots are functionally distinct. The dorsal roots contain **primary afferent neurones**, running from peripheral sensory receptors to the spinal cord and brain stem. The nerve cell bodies of these neurones are located in **dorsal root ganglia** (Fig. 8.5; see also Figs 1.8, 1.16), which appear as small enlargements on the dorsal roots near their convergence with the ventral roots at the entrance to the intervertebral foramina. The ventral roots of the spinal nerves carry **efferent neurones**, the cell bodies of which are located in the spinal grey matter. These are comprised of motor neurones, which innervate skeletal muscle, and preganglionic neurones of the autonomic nervous system.

The C1–C7 spinal nerves exit from the vertebral canal above the first seven cervical vertebrae; C8 spinal nerve exits

Spinous process of vertebra

Spinal cord

Transverse process

Arachnoid mater

Dorsal ramus of spinal nerve

Ventral ramus of spinal nerve

Dura mater

Dorsal root of spinal nerve

Dorsal root ganglion

Ventral root of spinal nerve

Vertebral body

Figure 8.1 **Transverse section through the thoracic region.** The diagram shows the relationship between the spinal cord, spinal nerves and vertebral column.

Spinal cord

Vertebral body

Intervertebral disc

Figure 8.2 **MR image of the vertebral column and spinal cord in the living subject.** (Courtesy of Professor A Jackson, Wolfson Molecular Imaging Centre, University of Manchester, Manchester, UK.)

below the seventh cervical vertebra and the remainder leave below their corresponding vertebrae (Fig. 8.3). Because of the different lengths of the spinal cord and the vertebral canal, only in the cervical region do the spinal cord segments lie adjacent to their corresponding vertebral bodies. Below this level, successive spinal nerve roots follow an increasingly oblique downwards course to reach their respective intervertebral foramina. This is most marked for

the lumbar and sacral roots, which descend below the termination of the cord in a leash-like arrangement, the **cauda equina** (Figs 8.3, 8.4).

Immediately after leaving the intervertebral foramina, spinal nerves divide to produce a thin **dorsal (posterior) ramus** and a much larger **ventral (anterior) ramus** (Fig. 8.1). The dorsal ramus supplies the muscles and skin of the back region. The ventral ramus supplies the muscles and skin of the front of the body and also the limbs.

The peripheral distribution of spinal nerves, including their pattern of cutaneous innervation (dermatomes) and innervation of muscle groups (myotomes) is described in Chapter 3.

Spinal meninges

The spinal cord, like the brain, is invested by three concentric meningeal coverings: the pia mater, arachnoid mater and dura mater (Figs 8.4, 8.5).

The innermost covering, the pia mater, is a delicate, vascular membrane that is closely applied to the surface of the cord and nerve roots. Along a line midway between the dorsal and ventral roots of the spinal nerves is attached a flat, membranous continuation of the pia, called the **denticulate ligament**. The ligament has a free lateral border for much of its length but, intermittently, lateral projections tether the spinal cord to the arachnoid, and through it to the dura.

Lumbar puncture and epidural anaesthesia

The lowest part of the spinal canal does not contain the spinal cord; consequently, hollow needles can be safely inserted into the subarachnoid space in order to remove CSF for diagnostic purposes (**lumbar puncture**) or to inject radio-opaque substances for the radiological delineation of the spinal canal and its contents (**myelography**). Similarly, anaesthetics may be introduced into the epidural space in surgical procedures (**epidural block**).

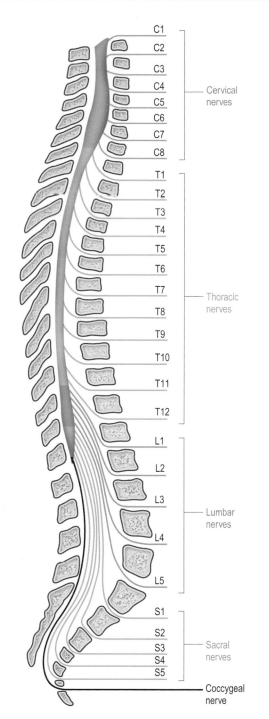

C1
C2
C3
C4
C5
C6
C7
C8

Cervical nerves

T1
T2
T3
T4
T5
T6
T7
T8
T9
T10
T11
T12

Thoracic nerves

L1
L2
L3
L4
L5

Lumbar nerves

S1
S2
S3
S4
S5

Sacral nerves

Coccygeal nerve

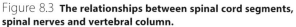

Figure 8.3 **The relationships between spinal cord segments, spinal nerves and vertebral column.**

Denticulate ligament

Dorsal roots of spinal nerves

Lumbar enlargement

Dura mater

Conus medullaris

Termination of the spinal cord at L1

Cauda equina

Epidural space

Filum terminale

Subarachnoid space

Termination of the subarachnoid space at S2

Figure 8.4 **Dorsal aspect of the spinal cord caudal to T9–T10.** The dura/arachnoid mater have been cut longitudinally and reflected to reveal the spinal cord and nerve roots within the subarachnoid space.

Figure 8.5 **Ventral aspect of the spinal cord, showing relationships of the spinal nerve roots and the meninges.**

Labels: Pia mater · Ventral root of spinal nerve · Denticulate ligament · Subarachnoid space · Spinal nerve · Arachnoid mater · Dura mater

---

Spinal nerve injury

The spinal nerve roots are vulnerable to compression by degenerative changes in the joints of the spinal column (**spondylosis**) and by **prolapse of intervertebral discs**. Prolapsed intervertebral discs in the cervical spine cause pain in the neck radiating to the arm and hand, accompanied by tingling sensations (paraesthesiae), weakness and wasting of the muscles corresponding to the radicular distribution, and numbness of the skin corresponding to the dermatomal distribution, together with loss of the tendon reflexes subserved by the particular root (Fig. 8.7). Similarly, lumbar prolapsed intervertebral discs lead to back pain and radiation of pain into the legs, known as **sciatica**. A large lumbosacral prolapsed disc may cause paralysis of the bladder and incontinence, demanding urgent neurosurgery.

The arachnoid mater lies between the pia and dura. It is a translucent membrane that invests the cord like a loose-fitting bag. Between the pia and arachnoid lies the subarachnoid space. This contains CSF, which is produced in the cerebral ventricular system (Ch. 6).

The outer covering of the cord, the dura mater, is a tough, fibrous membrane. It envelops the cord loosely, as does the arachnoid with which it is in contact, though separated by a theoretical plane, the **subdural space**. The dura is separated from the bony wall of the vertebral canal by the **epidural space**.

Although the spinal cord terminates at vertebral level L1–L2, the arachnoid and dural sheaths and, therefore, the subarachnoid space, continue caudally to S2. As the spinal nerve roots pass towards their intervertebral foramina they evaginate the arachnoid and dura, forming meningeal root sleeves that extend as far as the fusion of dorsal and ventral roots. Thereafter, the arachnoid and dura become continuous with the epineurium ensheathing the spinal nerve.

Figure 8.6 **Lateral aspect of the spinal column in the lumbar region, illustrating the intervertebral foramina and the emerging spinal nerves.**

Labels: Vertebral body · Spinal nerve · Intervertebral disc · Intervertebral foramen

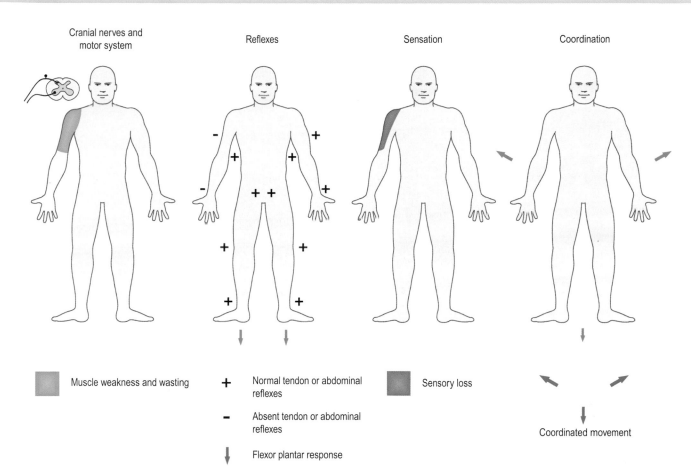

Figure 8.7 **Spinal nerve root lesion at the level of C5.**

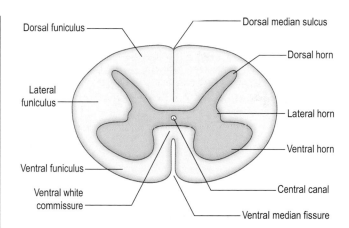

Figure 8.8 **Transverse section through the spinal cord showing the general disposition of grey and white matter.**

Internal structure of the spinal cord

The spinal cord is incompletely divided into two symmetrical halves by a **dorsal median sulcus** and a **ventral median fissure** (Fig. 8.8). In the centre of the cord is the small **central canal**, which is continuous rostrally with the cerebral ventricular system. Surrounding the central canal is the spinal **grey matter**, consisting of nerve cell bodies, their dendrites and synaptic contacts. The outer part of the cord consists of **white matter**, which contains ascending and descending nerve fibres. Some of these serve to join neighbouring and distant cord segments for the integration of their functions, while others run between the cord and the brain. Many of the fibres that share a common origin, course and termination are grouped together in fascicles, forming the long **tracts** of the spinal cord.

Different cord levels vary in the relative amounts and configuration of grey and white matter (Fig. 8.9). Higher levels contain greater amounts of white matter. This is because ascending tracts gain fibres at each successive level, whereas the opposite is true of descending tracts.

Grey matter of the spinal cord

The grey matter is approximately H-shaped, or butterfly-shaped, with four protrusions, the **dorsal (posterior)** and

Figure 8.10 **Lamination of spinal grey matter (Rexed's laminae).**

Figure 8.9 **Transverse sections through the spinal cord at (A) cervical, (B) thoracic, (C) lumbar and (D) sacral levels.** The histological method employed (Weigert–Pal) stains white matter (myelinated nerve fibres), leaving grey matter (nerve cell bodies) relatively unstained.

ventral **(anterior) horns**, extending dorso- and ventrolaterally towards the attachment zones of the dorsal and ventral root fascicles, respectively. The size and shape of the dorsal and ventral horns varies according to the level (Fig. 8.9). Many afferent nerve fibres entering in the dorsal roots terminate in the dorsal horn, while the ventral horn contains the cell bodies of motor neurones that exit through the ventral nerve roots and innervate skeletal muscle. Both dorsal and ventral horns are, therefore, particularly well developed at cervical and lumbar levels in association with innervation of the upper and lower limbs. Thoracic and upper lumbar segments additionally possess a small **lateral or intermediolateral horn**, located between the dorsal and ventral horns, which contains the cell bodies of **preganglionic sympathetic neurones** (Figs 8.8, 8.9B).

The grey matter of the spinal cord may be divided, on the basis of its cytoarchitecture, into ten zones, known as **Rexed's laminae**, which are numbered sequentially from dorsal to ventral (Fig. 8.10). Some of these laminae are equated with cell groupings of particular functional types.

Dorsal horn

Afferent fibres entering through the dorsal roots divide into ascending and descending branches. They mostly terminate near their point of entry but may travel for varying distances in either direction, running in the **dorsolateral fasciculus** or **Lissauer's tract**, which is located superficial to the tip of the dorsal horn (see Fig. 8.14). Dorsal root afferents may, therefore, establish synaptic contacts over several segments of spinal grey matter. Dorsal root fibres terminate extensively within the grey matter but most densely in the dorsal horn. Cutaneous afferents tend to terminate in superficial (dorsal) laminae, while proprioceptive and muscle afferents project mostly to deeper laminae.

The tip of the dorsal horn, approximating to Rexed's laminae I–III, is also known as the **substantia gelatinosa**. This region receives collaterals of the smallest-diameter myelinated (group A delta) and unmyelinated (group C) afferents that are associated with nociception. These neurones are excitatory and use glutamic acid and the peptide substance P as neurotransmitters. In the substantia gelatinosa, complex interactions occur with other types of afferent terminal, interneurones, and with descending pathways from the brain, which control the transmission of pain information to ascending spinothalamic and spinoreticular tract neurones distributed throughout the dorsal horn. For example, input from large-diameter afferents carrying tactile information inhibits transmission of nociceptive impulses to ascending tract neurones, which explains why rubbing a sore spot can relieve pain.

The substantia gelatinosa contains high levels of the endogenous opioid peptide enkephalin, which is thought to act as a transmitter of some dorsal horn interneurones. These establish presynaptic contacts with the terminals of primary afferent neurones that possess opiate receptors. Occupation of these receptors decreases the release of substance P. The analgesic properties of opiates such as morphine are partly a result of their action at this site. The complex interactions between afferent nerve terminals, spinal interneurones and descending pathways, that together regulate the transmission of nociceptive information to ascending spinothalamic and spinoreticular tract fibres, constitute what is referred to as the 'gate control theory' of pain.

Deeper in the dorsal horn, lamina VII contains a number of important cell groups. At cord levels C8–L3 lie the cells of **Clarke's column** (thoracic nucleus, nucleus dorsalis), which are the origin of ascending fibres of the dorsal spinocerebellar tract. The cells of Clarke's column receive afferent input from muscle spindles, Golgi tendon organs, tactile and pressure receptors. At thoracic and upper lumbar levels, the lateral part of lamina VII also contains preganglionic sympathetic neurones that constitute the lateral horn, while at sacral levels (S2–S4) it contains preganglionic parasympathetic neurones.

Ventral horn

In the ventral horn, lamina IX corresponds to groups of motor neurones that innervate skeletal muscle. These are of two types:

1. **Alpha motor neurones**, which innervate extrafusal muscle fibres
2. **Gamma motor neurones**, which innervate intrafusal muscle fibres (within muscle spindles).

The ventral horn is particularly well developed in the cervical and lumbar enlargements owing to the presence of motor neurones innervating the upper and lower limbs. Generally speaking, neurones innervating axial musculature (neck and trunk) tend to be located medially, while those innervating limb muscles are positioned more laterally. In the ventral horn of cord segments C3–C5 is located the **phrenic nucleus**, a group of motor neurones that innervate the diaphragm via the phrenic nerve and are, thus, essential for breathing. Cells in the ventral horn receive direct input from certain dorsal root afferents (e.g. from muscle spindles for mediation of the stretch reflex). Importantly, they also receive input from pathways descending from higher centres concerned with motor control.

Motor neuronopathies

The lower motor neurones of the spinal cord may be selectively affected by two diseases.

Poliomyelitis is an acute viral infection of the neurones leading to rapid paralysis and wasting of the limb and respiratory muscles. The disability is often asymmetrical and frequently affects the legs. Recovery occurs but may be incomplete.

Motor neurone disease is a chronic degenerative disorder that affects both lower motor neurones and the descending tracts to the spinal cord (upper motor neurones). Degeneration of ventral horn cells causes weakness, wasting, hypotonia and fasciculation of the limb muscles (**progressive muscular atrophy**). Degeneration of descending pathways leads to weakness and spasticity of the limb muscles (**amyotrophic lateral sclerosis**).

sense (e.g. in delay, duration and extent) as a result of intersegmental and supraspinal influences.

Anatomically, the pathways mediating reflex actions consist of afferent neurones conveying impulses from sensory receptors to the CNS (spinal cord or brain stem) and efferent neurones running from the CNS to the effector organ (muscle or gland). In all but the simplest reflexes, interneurones within the CNS are interposed between the afferent and efferent components. The internal organisation of the spinal cord (and brain stem) thus subserves a number of more or less complex reflex functions, some of which are both relatively well understood and clinically important.

Stretch reflex

If a muscle is stretched, it responds by contracting, and this is known as the **stretch** or **myotatic reflex**. Anatomically, this is the simplest of reflexes and is mediated by a **monosynaptic reflex arc** (Fig. 8.11). It consists of afferent neurones that convey impulses from muscle stretch receptors to the CNS and motor neurones that convey impulses back to the stretched muscle.

Stretch receptors within muscles consist of sensory nerve endings that attach to the central, non-contractile region of specialised muscle cells called **intrafusal muscle fibres** (see also Ch. 3). Intrafusal muscle fibres are oriented parallel to the long axis of the main muscle and occur in groups called **muscle spindles**. Stretch applied to the muscle in which they lie stimulates the sensory endings. Their afferent fibres carry impulses to the CNS, where they make monosynaptic excitatory contact with alpha motor neurones that innervate the bulk of the muscle (**extrafusal muscle fibres**) and make it contract.

There are two types of intrafusal muscle fibre: **nuclear bag** and **nuclear chain** fibres. These bear two types of sensory ending:

1. **Primary or annulospiral endings**, associated with group Ia afferent fibres,
2. **Secondary** or **flower-spray endings**, associated with group II afferents.

When a muscle is stretched, these endings are stimulated. Primary endings have both velocity and length sensitivity, while secondary endings have essentially only length

---

Grey matter of the spinal cord

- Internally, the spinal cord consists of a central core of grey matter (cell bodies) and an outer mantle of white matter (nerve fibres).
- Within the grey matter, the dorsal horn is the main site of termination of primary afferent fibres. It includes the substantia gelatinosa, which is important in transmission of nociceptive impulses to the brain.
- The lateral horn contains preganglionic sympathetic neurones.
- The ventral horn contains alpha and gamma motor neurones, also known as lower motor neurones.

Spinal reflexes

A reflex is an involuntary, stereotyped pattern of response brought about by a sensory stimulus. Although the qualitative nature of an established reflex response is constant, it may vary considerably in a quantitative

Figure 8.11 **The stretch reflex and reciprocal innervation. (A)** The quadriceps stretch reflex is illustrated, whereby striking the patellar tendon elicits extension of the knee; **(B)** Reciprocal innervation. While stretching of the quadriceps muscle causes its reflex contraction, the motor neurones of antagonistic muscles (knee flexors) are inhibited by interneuronal connection within the spinal cord.

sensitivity. Group Ia afferents from a particular muscle make excitatory monosynaptic contact with alpha motor neurones innervating the same muscle and, thus, mediate the myotatic reflex.

Stretch reflexes are important in the control of skeletal muscle tone, which refers to the degree of resistance to passive movement and is determined by the proportion of motor units that are active at any one time. When the upper motor neurones are damaged, muscle tone is increased during initial muscle stretch (spasticity). Since stretch reflexes operate to maintain muscles at a constant length in opposition to imposed stretch, they are important in the control of posture. By their action, activity is maintained in neck, trunk and lower limb extensor muscles (anti-gravity muscles) that support an upright body posture against the force of gravity and are stretched when these body parts become flexed.

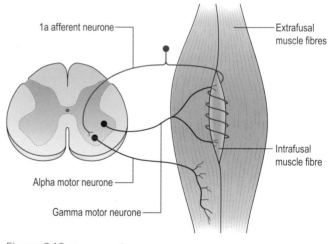

Figure 8.12 **Gamma reflex loop.**

In addition to alpha motor neurones, which innervate extrafusal muscle fibres, the ventral horn of the spinal cord (and motor cranial nerve nuclei) contain **gamma motor neurones**, which innervate the polar, contractile elements of intrafusal muscle fibres (Fig. 8.12). When gamma motor neurones are activated, the resultant contraction of the intrafusal muscle fibre applies tension to the sensory endings. This lowers the threshold of the stretch receptors to externally applied stretch and, thus, increases the sensitivity of the stretch reflex (the **gamma reflex loop**, Fig. 8.12).

Like alpha motor neurones, gamma motor neurones are under the influence of descending pathways from the brain. Abnormalities in the activity of these pathways, therefore, which occur in many pathological conditions, induce

Tendon reflexes

Deep tendon reflexes, or tendon jerks, are monosynaptic stretch reflexes elicited during clinical examination by percussion of the tendon of the muscle by a tendon hammer. Each tendon reflex is subserved by certain spinal cord segments:

Reflex	Cord segments
Biceps reflex (biceps jerk)	C5/C6
Brachioradialis reflex (supinator jerk)	C5/C6
Triceps reflex (triceps jerk)	C6/C7
Quadriceps reflex (knee jerk)	L3/L4
Achilles tendon reflex (ankle jerk)	S1/S2

changes in the sensitivity of stretch reflexes. This is evidenced by abnormalities in muscle tone.

When a stretch reflex is elicited (e.g. the quadriceps reflex, by tapping the patellar tendon), primary afferent fibres from the muscle spindle excite not only the alpha motor neurones of the stretched muscle but also interneurones that inhibit the alpha motor neurones of antagonistic muscles (e.g. the knee flexors, Fig. 8.11). This illustrates the general principle of **reciprocal innervation** of agonist and antagonist muscle groups.

Flexor reflex

Noxious cutaneous stimulation of the limbs causes withdrawal from the offending stimulus. This is mediated by **a polysynaptic reflex** in which one or more interneurones are interposed between afferent and efferent neurones. Primary afferent fibres activate interneurones within the spinal grey matter, which in turn excite alpha motor neurones innervating the limb flexor muscles (Fig. 8.13). Flexion of a limb about several joints requires the coordinated action of more than one spinal segment and this is achieved by collateralisation of primary afferents and interneurones.

All forms of cutaneous stimulation have the potential to elicit the flexor reflex, but this is normally prevented by descending pathways from the brain unless the stimulus is painful. In certain pathological conditions, the descending inhibitory influence is lost and even innocuous cutaneous stimulation can cause limb withdrawal. The extensor plantar response (Babinski reflex) is characterised by extension (dorsiflexion) of the great toe and splaying of the other toes in response to stimulation of the sole of the foot.

Physiologically, it is a flexor reflex and is present in infants before myelination of the corticospinal tract has taken place. Thereafter, the reflex is absent, being suppressed by descending corticospinal influences (stimulation of the sole of the foot then causing a flexor plantar response, with curling of the toes). When the descending influence is lost (e.g. following a stroke in the internal capsule) the extensor plantar reflex re-emerges. It is regarded as pathonomic of damage to the corticospinal tract.

Activation of the flexor reflex in a weight-bearing limb (e.g. by standing on a pin) simultaneously causes reflex extension of the contralateral limb to take the weight of the body. This is called the **crossed extensor reflex** (Fig. 8.13). It is mediated by axon collaterals which cross the midline of the cord and excite the alpha motor neurones of contralateral limb extensor muscles.

Spinal reflexes

- The internal organisation of the cord subserves a number of important reflex functions.
- The monosynaptic stretch reflex mediates muscle contraction in response to stretch of muscle spindles.
- The sensitivity of the stretch reflex is regulated by gamma motor neurones, which provide motor innervation to the spindle fibres.
- The stretch reflex is responsible for maintenance of muscle tone and is clinically tested as the deep tendon reflexes.
- The polysynaptic flexor reflex mediates limb withdrawal from noxious stimuli.

Figure 8.13 **Flexor reflex and crossed extensor reflex.**

White matter of the spinal cord

The grey matter of the spinal cord is completely surrounded by white matter, which consists of ascending and descending nerve fibres. The white matter is sometimes considered to be divided into dorsal, lateral and ventral columns or **funiculi** (Fig. 8.8). Nerve fibres sharing common origins, terminations and functions are organised into **tracts** or **fasciculi** (Latin for small bundles). Some fibres interconnect adjacent or distant cord segments and permit intersegmental coordination, while other fibres are longer and serve to join the spinal cord with the brain. The **intersegmental**, or **propriospinal**, fibres occupy a narrow band immediately peripheral to the grey matter. This is known as the **fasciculus proprius** (Fig. 8.14). Nerve fibres running between the spinal cord and the brain constitute the **ascending** and **descending tracts** of the spinal cord (Figs 8.14–8.20).

Ascending spinal tracts

Ascending tracts carry impulses from pain, thermal, tactile, muscle and joint receptors to the brain. Some of this information eventually reaches a conscious level (the cerebral cortex), while some is destined for subconscious centres (e.g. the cerebellum).

Pathways that carry information to a conscious level share certain common characteristics.

There is a sequence of three neurones between the peripheral receptor and the cerebral cortex.

- The first neurone (first-order neurone or primary afferent neurone) enters the spinal cord through the dorsal root of a spinal nerve and its cell body lies in the dorsal root ganglion. The central process may collateralise extensively and make synaptic connections that mediate spinal reflexes and intersegmental coordination. The main fibre remains on the ipsilateral side of the cord and terminates in synaptic contact with the second neurone either in the spinal grey matter or in the medulla oblongata of the brain stem, depending on the modality.

- The second neurone (second-order neurone) has its cell body in the cord or medulla oblongata. Its axon crosses over (decussates) to the opposite side of the CNS and ascends to the thalamus, where it terminates upon the third neurone.

- The third neurone (third-order neurone) has its cell body in the thalamus. Its axon passes to the somatosensory cortex in the parietal lobe of the ipsilateral cerebral hemisphere.

Two main tract systems in the spinal cord fit into this pattern: the dorsal (posterior) columns and the spinothalamic tracts.

Dorsal columns

The dorsal columns are located between the dorsal median sulcus and the dorsal horn. Two tracts are recognised: **the fasciculus gracilis**, situated medially and **the fasciculus cuneatus**, situated laterally. The tracts carry impulses concerned with proprioception (movement and joint position sense) and discriminative (fine) touch.

The dorsal columns contain the axons of primary afferent neurones that have entered the cord through the dorsal roots of spinal nerves (Fig. 8.15). The fasciculus gracilis consists of fibres that join the cord at sacral, lumbar and lower thoracic levels and, thus, includes those from the lower limb. Fibres of the fasciculus cuneatus enter via the upper thoracic and cervical dorsal roots and, thus, include those from the upper limb. Since the dorsal columns contain primary afferent neurones, they carry information relating to the ipsilateral side of the body. Fibres ascend without interruption to the medulla oblongata where they terminate upon second-order neurones, the cell bodies of which are located in the **nucleus gracilis** and **nucleus cuneatus** (see also p. 92).

Ascending tracts — Descending tracts

Fasciculus gracilis
Fasciculus cuneatus
Dorsal spinocerebellar tract
Ventral spinocerebellar tract
Spinothalamic tract

Fasciculus proprius
Lissauer's tract
Lateral corticospinal tract
Rubrospinal tract
Medial longitudinal fasciculus
Medullary reticulospinal tract
Lateral vestibulospinal tract
Pontine reticulospinal tract
Tectospinal tract
Ventral corticospinal tract

Figure 8.14 **Ascending and descending tracts of the spinal cord.** All ascending and descending tracts are present bilaterally. In this figure, ascending tracts are emphasised on the left side and descending tracts are emphasised on the right side. In addition, the location of Lissauer's tract and the fasciculus proprius (which contain both ascending and descending fibres) are shown.

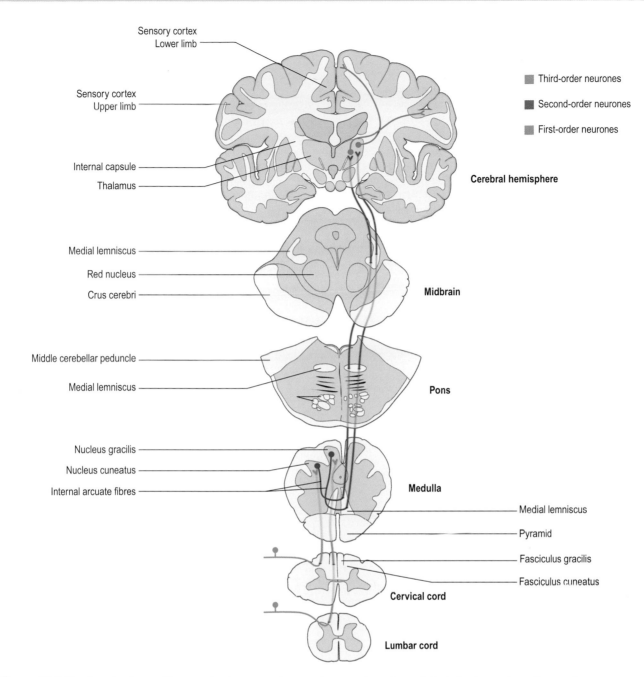

Figure 8.15 **The dorsal columns.** The central pathways carrying conscious proprioception and discriminative touch are illustrated.

The axons of the second-order neurones decussate in the medulla as **internal arcuate fibres** and, thereafter, ascend through the brain stem as the **medial lemniscus**. The medial lemniscus terminates in the **ventral posterior** (**VP**) **nucleus** of the thalamus upon third-order thalamocortical neurones. These in turn project to the somatosensory cortex, located in the postcentral gyrus of the parietal lobe.

Lesions of the dorsal columns

Tabes dorsalis is a late manifestation of syphilitic infection of the CNS. It chiefly affects the lumbosacral dorsal spinal roots and the dorsal columns of the spinal cord. The loss of proprioception leads to a high steppage and unsteady gait (**sensory ataxia**), which is exacerbated when the eyes are closed (**Romberg's sign**).

Subacute combined degeneration of the spinal cord is a systemic disease resulting from a deficiency of vitamin B_{12} (cyanocobalamin), which also causes pernicious anaemia. The degeneration of the dorsal columns produces sensory ataxia. The lateral columns of the spinal cord are also involved (combined), causing weakness and spasticity of the limbs. The disorder, although uncommon, is an important one since proper treatment with vitamin B_{12} can lead to complete recovery.

In **multiple sclerosis**, an immune disease, specific damage to the fasciculus cuneatus of the cervical spinal cord leads to loss of proprioception in the hands and fingers, causing profound loss of dexterity and inability to identify the shape and nature of objects by touch alone (**astereognosis**).

Spinothalamic tract

The spinothalamic tract lies lateral and ventral to the ventral horn of the spinal grey matter. It carries information related to pain and thermal sensations and also non-discriminative (course) touch and pressure. Some authorities identify distinct lateral and ventral spinothalamic tracts conveying pain and temperature or touch and pressure, respectively, but fibres carrying these modalities are probably intermingled to some extent.

The spinothalamic tract contains second-order neurones, the cell bodies of which lie in the contralateral dorsal horn and receive input from primary afferent fibres that terminate in this region (Fig. 8.16). After leaving the parent cell bodies, spinothalamic axons decussate to the opposite side of the cord by passing through the **ventral white commissure**, which lies ventral to the central canal of the cord, and, thus,

enter the contralateral spinothalamic tract. Axons carrying pain and temperature decussate promptly within one segment of their origin, while those carrying touch and pressure may ascend for several segments before crossing.

In the brain stem, the spinothalamic fibres run in close proximity to the medial lemniscus and are known as the **spinal lemniscus**. The majority of fibres terminate in the ventral posterior nucleus of the thalamus, contacting third-order thalamocortical neurones that project to the somatosensory cortex.

The spinothalamic tract is sometimes referred to as the neospinothalamic system. It is highly organised somatotopically; consequently, the origin of sensory stimuli can be accurately localised. It is thought to be the route via which sharp, pricking pain (sometimes called 'fast' pain) is conducted.

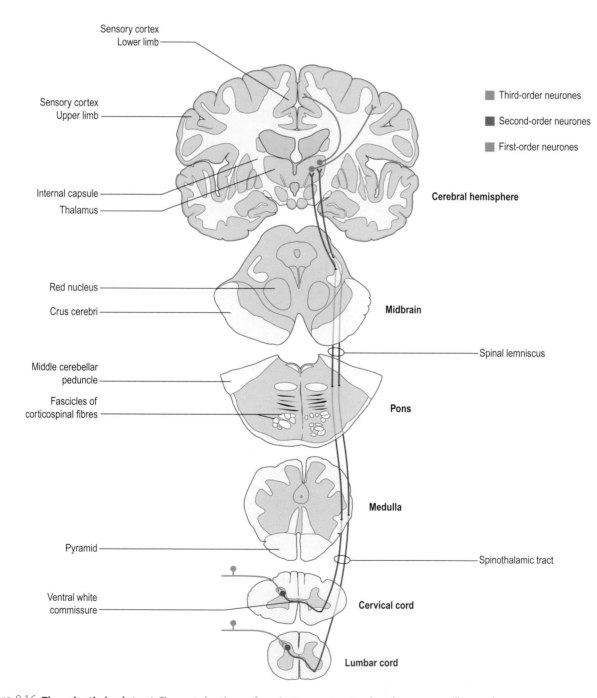

Figure 8.16 **The spinothalamic tract.** The central pathways for pain, temperature, touch and pressure are illustrated.

Spinothalamic tract lesions

The spinothalamic tracts can be selectively damaged in **syringomyelia**, in which the central canal becomes enlarged to form a cavity compressing adjacent nerve fibres. The second-order neurones subserving pain and temperature are damaged as they decussate in the ventral white commissure, close to the central canal, causing a selective loss of pain and temperature awareness in the upper limbs. This is termed a **dissociated sensory loss**, since light touch and proprioceptive sensation are retained. The patient injures and burns the hands painlessly, and the joints of the limbs become disorganised without discomfort (**Charcot's joints**).

Selective surgical destruction of the spinothalamic tracts (**cordotomy** or **tractotomy**) is sometimes performed for the neurosurgical relief of intractable pain from a variety of causes.

Friedreich's ataxia

Friedreich's ataxia is an inherited degenerative disease in which the spinocerebellar tracts are particularly disordered, leading to profound incoordination of the arms (intention tremor) and a wide-based, reeling gait (ataxia). The disorder begins in childhood and the patient is wheelchair-bound by 20 years of age.

The **spinoreticulothalamic system** represents an additional, phylogenetically older, route by which nociceptive sensory impulses ascend to higher centres. Some second-order neurones arising from the dorsal horn ascend in the ventrolateral region of the cord and then terminate in the brain stem reticular formation, particularly within the medulla. Reticulothalamic fibres then ascend to the intralaminar thalamic nuclei, which in turn activate the cerebral cortex. The spinoreticulothalamic system is poorly organised somatotopically and is thought to be the route via which dull, aching pain (sometimes called 'slow' pain) is transmitted to a conscious level. Activation of spinothalamic and spinoreticular fibres, which may ultimately be perceived as unpleasant or painful, can be modulated by descending pathways from the brain.

Ascending pathways that carry impulses to a subconscious level are represented principally by the spinocerebellar tracts.

Spinocerebellar tracts

Fibres of the ascending spinocerebellar tracts form dorsal and ventral tracts that are located near the dorsolateral and ventrolateral surfaces of the cord, respectively. Both tracts carry information derived from muscle spindles, Golgi tendon organs and tactile receptors to the cerebellum for the control of posture and coordination of movement.

The spinocerebellar system consists of a sequence of only two neurones. Both spinocerebellar tracts contain second-order neurones whose cell bodies of origin lie in the base of the dorsal horn; they receive input from primary afferent fibres terminating in this region. The tract neurones terminate directly in the cerebellar cortex, predominantly within the vermis. Fibres of the dorsal spinocerebellar tract originate from a prominent group of cells known as **Clarke's column**. The axons ascend ipsilaterally to enter the cerebellum through the **inferior cerebellar peduncle**. Fibres of the ventral spinocerebellar tract decussate, ascend on the contralateral side of the cord and enter the cerebellum via the **superior cerebellar peduncle**. Some axons then re-cross within the cerebellar white matter.

White matter of the spinal cord: principal ascending tracts

- Ascending tracts carry afferent information to conscious and subconscious levels. Pathways to a conscious level follow a basic plan of three neurones in a chain from peripheral receptor to cerebral cortex.
- Dorsal columns (fasciculus gracilis and cuneatus) carry proprioception and discriminative touch. They convey first-order neurones ipsilaterally to the nuclei gracilis and cuneatus of the medulla. Second-order neurones decussate and pass to the thalamus. Third-order neurones project to the somatosensory cortex. Lesions (e.g. tabes dorsalis, vitamin B_{12} deficiency) lead to ataxia and loss of discriminative touch.
- Spinothalamic tract carries pain, temperature, touch and pressure. The tract contains second-order neurones with cell bodies in the dorsal horn. Axons decussate and pass to the thalamus. Third-order neurones project to the somatosensory cortex. Lesions (e.g. syringomyelia) lead to impairment of pain, temperature, touch and pressure sensitivity on the contralateral side.
- Dorsal and ventral spinocerebellar tracts contain second-order neurones carrying muscle, joint and tactile information involved in motor control. Lesions lead to ataxia (e.g. Friedreich's ataxia).

Descending spinal tracts

Descending tracts of the spinal cord (Fig. 8.14) originate from the cerebral cortex and brain stem. They are concerned with the control of movement, muscle tone, spinal reflexes, spinal autonomic functions and the modulation of sensory transmission to higher centres.

Corticospinal tracts

The corticospinal tracts (Fig. 8.17) are particularly concerned with the control of voluntary, discrete, skilled movements, especially those of the distal parts of the limbs. Such movements are sometimes referred to as 'fractionated' movements. Corticospinal tract neurones arise from cell bodies in the cerebral cortex. The cells of origin are widely distributed in the motor and sensory cortices, including the **precentral gyrus** or **primary motor cortex**, where the large **Betz cells** give rise to the largest diameter corticospinal axons. Corticospinal axons leave the cerebral hemispheres by passing through the massive subcortical fibre systems of the **corona radiata** and **internal capsule** to enter the **crus cerebri** of the midbrain.

Having passed through the ventral portion of the pons, corticospinal fibres reach the medulla oblongata, where they form two prominent columns on the ventral surface. These are called the **pyramids** and for this reason the term

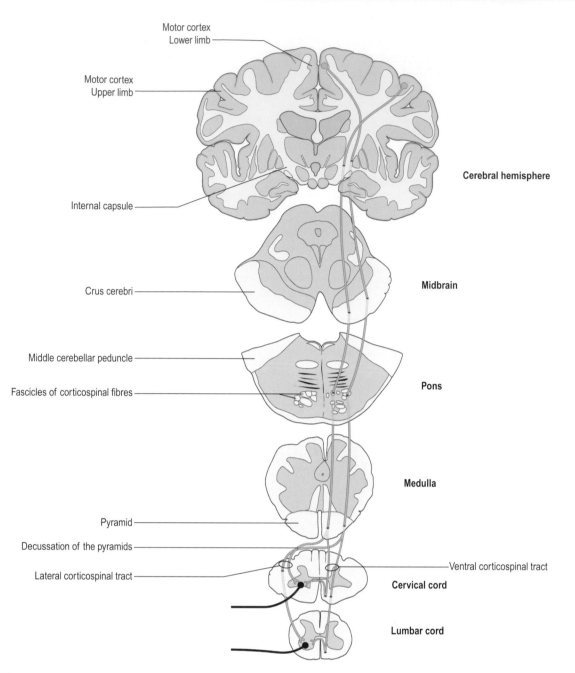

Motor cortex
Lower limb

Motor cortex
Upper limb

Cerebral hemisphere

Internal capsule

Crus cerebri

Midbrain

Middle cerebellar peduncle

Fascicles of corticospinal fibres

Pons

Medulla

Pyramid

Decussation of the pyramids

Ventral corticospinal tract

Lateral corticospinal tract

Cervical cord

Lumbar cord

Figure 8.17 **Corticospinal tracts.**

pyramidal tract is used as an alternative name for the corticospinal tract. In the caudal medulla, the fibres of the pyramids undergo subtotal decussation. About 75–90% of fibres decussate and enter the contralateral **lateral corticospinal tract**, which is located in the lateral part of the spinal white matter, deep to the dorsal spinocerebellar

Hereditary spastic paraparesis
Hereditary spastic paraparesis is an inherited degenerative disorder (autosomal dominant) in which progressive weakness affects the legs, leading to marked stiffness of gait. Degeneration of the lateral columns, including the lateral corticospinal tract, chiefly affects the thoracic spinal cord, causing a spastic paraparesis with hyperreflexia and extensor plantar responses, but with sparing of sensation and bladder function.

tract; 10–25% of pyramidal fibres remain ipsilateral and enter the **ventral corticospinal tract** located lateral to the ventral median fissure. They also decussate near to their termination; as a result, the fibres of the pyramidal tract effectively innervate the contralateral side of the spinal cord. Approximately 55% of corticospinal neurones terminate at cervical levels, 20% at thoracic and 25% at lumbosacral levels. Fibres terminate extensively in the spinal grey matter. Many of those fibres that originate from the motor cortex terminate in the ventral horn, some making monosynaptic contact with motor neurones.

Rubrospinal tract
The rubrospinal tract originates from the **red nucleus** of the midbrain tegmentum (Fig. 8.18). It exerts control over the tone of limb flexor muscles, being excitatory to the motor neurones of these muscles. Axons leaving the cells of the red nucleus course ventromedially and cross in the **ventral tegmental decussation**, after which they descend

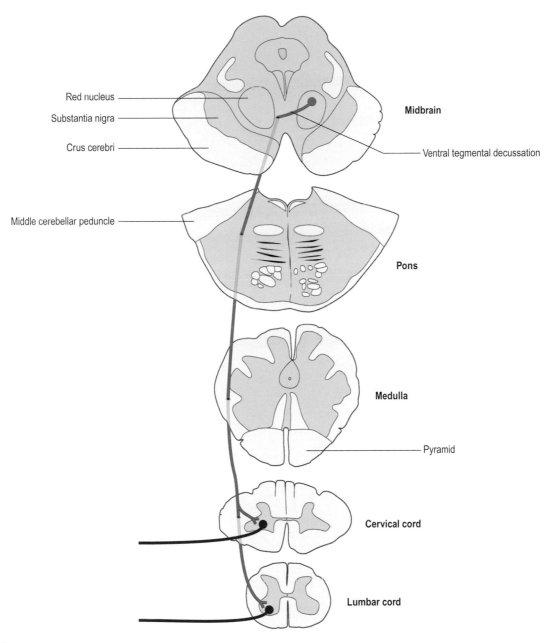

Red nucleus

Substantia nigra

Crus cerebri

Midbrain

Ventral tegmental decussation

Middle cerebellar peduncle

Pons

Medulla

Pyramid

Cervical cord

Lumbar cord

Figure 8.18 **Rubrospinal tract.**

to the spinal cord where they lie ventrolateral to, and partly intermingled with, the lateral corticospinal tract.

The red nucleus receives afferent fibres from the motor cortex and from the cerebellum. The rubrospinal tract, therefore, represents a non-pyramidal route by which the motor cortex and cerebellum can influence spinal motor activity.

Tectospinal tract

Tectospinal fibres arise from the **superior colliculus** of the midbrain (Fig. 8.19). Axons pass ventromedially around the periaqueductal grey matter and cross in the **dorsal tegmental decussation**. In the spinal cord, descending tectospinal fibres lie near the ventral median fissure and terminate predominantly in cervical segments. The superior colliculus receives visual input and the tectospinal tract is thought to mediate reflex movements in response to visual stimuli.

Vestibulospinal tracts

Vestibulospinal fibres arise from the **vestibular nuclei** situated in the pons and medulla, in and near the floor of the fourth ventricle (Fig. 8.20). The vestibular nuclei receive input from the labyrinthine system by way of the vestibular nerve and from the cerebellum.

Axons from cells of the **lateral vestibular nucleus (Deiters' nucleus)** descend ipsilaterally as the **lateral vestibulospinal tract**, which is located in the ventral funiculus. Lateral vestibulospinal tract fibres mediate excitatory influences upon extensor motor neurones. They serve to control extensor muscle tone in the anti-gravity maintenance of posture.

The **medial vestibular nucleus** contributes descending fibres to the ipsilateral **medial longitudinal fasciculus**, also known as the **medial vestibulospinal tract**, which is located adjacent to the ventral median fissure.

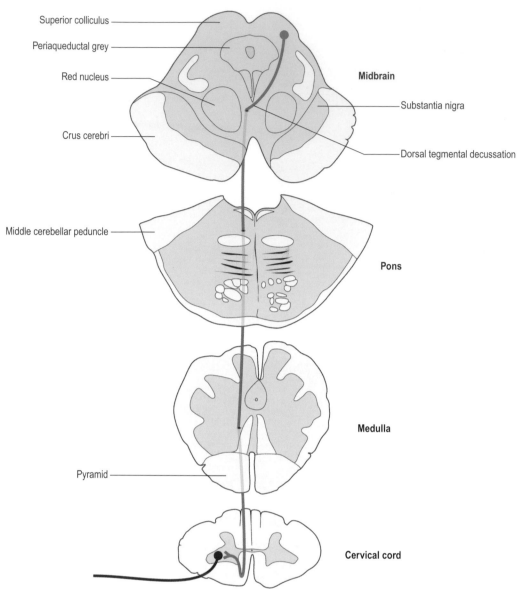

Superior colliculus
Periaqueductal grey
Red nucleus
Crus cerebri
Middle cerebellar peduncle
Pyramid

Midbrain
Substantia nigra
Dorsal tegmental decussation

Pons

Medulla

Cervical cord

Figure 8.19 **Tectospinal tract.**

Reticulospinal tracts

The reticular formation of the pons and medulla gives rise to reticulospinal fibres. Axons arising from the pontine reticular formation descend ipsilaterally as the **medial (or pontine) reticulospinal tract**. Axons from the medulla descend bilaterally in the **lateral (or medullary) reticulospinal tracts**. Both tracts are located in the ventral funiculus.

Reticulospinal fibres influence voluntary movement, reflex activity and muscle tone by controlling the activity of both alpha and gamma motor neurones. They also mediate pressor and depressor effects upon the circulatory system and are involved in the control of breathing.

White matter of the spinal cord: principal descending tracts

- Corticospinal tract controls discrete, skilled movements, particularly of the distal extremities. It originates from motor and sensory cortices. Fibres descend through the internal capsule, crus cerebri and ventral pons to reach the medullary pyramid. Most fibres (75–90%) decussate to form the lateral corticospinal tract, the remainder forming the ventral corticospinal tract.
- Rubrospinal tract controls limb flexor muscles and originates from the red nucleus of the midbrain. Fibres cross in the ventral tegmental decussation.
- Tectospinal tract is involved in reflex responses to visual input. It originates from the contralateral superior colliculus and fibres cross in the dorsal tegmental decussation.
- Vestibulospinal tracts descend from the vestibular nuclei. The lateral tract originates from the ipsilateral lateral vestibular nucleus and mediates excitation of limb extensor muscles.
- Reticulospinal tracts descend from the pons and medulla. They are involved in the control of reflex activities, muscle tone and vital functions.

Figure 8.20 **Vestibulospinal tracts.**

Lesions of the spinal cord

Focal lesions of the spinal cord and the nerve roots produce clinical manifestations in two ways:

1. The lesion destroys function at the segmental level.

2. The lesion interrupts descending motor and ascending sensory tracts.

Damage to different parts of the spinal cord, therefore, is accompanied by distinctive clinical syndromes (Fig. 8.21).

Figure 8.21 **(A) Upper cervical cord lesion.** A high cervical cord lesion causes spastic tetraplegia with hyperreflexia, extensor plantar responses (upper motor neurone lesion), incontinence, sensory loss below the level of the lesion and 'sensory' ataxia. **(B) Lower cervical cord lesion.** A lower cervical cord lesion causes weakness, wasting and fasciculation of muscles, and areflexia of the upper limbs (lower motor neurone lesion). In addition, there is spastic paraparesis, hyperreflexia and extensor plantar responses (upper motor neurone lesion) in the lower limbs, incontinence, sensory loss below the level of the lesion and 'sensory' ataxia.

Figure 8.21 Continued **(C) Thoracic cord lesion.** A thoracic cord lesion causes a spastic paraparesis, hyperreflexia and extensor plantar responses (upper motor neurone lesion), incontinence, sensory loss below the level of the lesion and 'sensory' ataxia. **(D) Lumbar cord lesion.** A lumbar cord lesion causes weakness, wasting and fasciculation of muscles, areflexia of the lower limbs (lower motor neurone lesion), incontinence, sensory loss below the level of the lesion and 'sensory' ataxia.

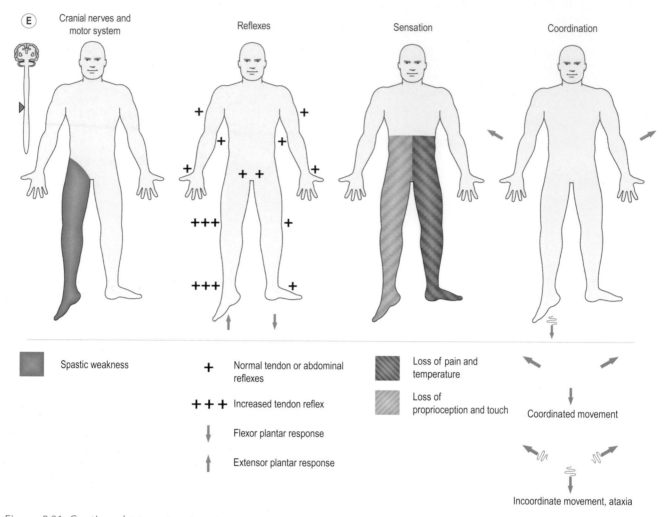

Figure 8.21 Continued **(E) Hemisection of the cord gives rise to the Brown–Séquard syndrome.** This is characterised by ipsilateral loss of proprioception and upper motor neurone signs (hemiplegia/monoplegia) plus contralateral loss of pain and temperature sensation.

Chapter 9
Brain stem

The brain stem consists of the medulla oblongata, pons and midbrain. The archaic term 'bulb' is applied to the brain stem in compound anatomical names given to nerve fibres originating from, or terminating in, the brain stem (e.g. 'corticobulbar' refers to axons that arise in the cerebral cortex and terminate in the brain stem). It is also used clinically to denote the medulla in such terms as 'bulbar palsy' and 'pseudobulbar palsy', which describe syndromes associated with medullary dysfunction.

The brain stem lies upon the basal portion of the occipital bone (clivus) and is connected to, and largely covered by, the cerebellum. Caudally, the medulla is continuous with the spinal cord just below the foramen magnum. Rostrally, the midbrain is continuous with the diencephalon of the forebrain.

The brain stem contains numerous ascending and descending fibre tracts. Some of these pass throughout its whole length, having their origin in the spinal cord or cerebral hemisphere, respectively; others have their origin or termination within brain stem nuclei. Certain of these brain stem nuclei receive fibres from, or send fibres into, cranial nerves, 10 pairs of which (III–XII) attach to the surface of the brain stem. These are known as the **cranial nerve nuclei**. In addition, the brain stem contains a complex and heterogeneous matrix of neurones known as the **reticular formation**, within which a number of individually identified nuclei exist. The reticular formation has several important functions, including control over the level of consciousness, the perception of pain and regulation of the cardiovascular and respiratory systems. It also has extensive connections with the cranial nerve nuclei, with the cerebellum, and with brain stem and spinal motor mechanisms, through which it influences movement, posture and muscle tone.

External features of the brain stem

Dorsal surface of the brain stem
The dorsal surface of the brain stem can be viewed if the overlying cerebellum is removed by cutting the three pairs of nerve fibre bundles, or **peduncles**, by which it is attached on each side (Figs 9.1, 9.2). On the dorsal surface of the medulla, the midline is marked by a dorsal median sulcus, continuous with that of the spinal cord. In the caudal part of the medulla, the **dorsal columns (fasciculi gracilis** and **cuneatus**, containing first-order sensory neurones) continue rostrally from the spinal cord to their termination in the **nuclei gracilis** and **cuneatus**, the locations of which are marked by two small elevations, the gracile and cuneate tubercles.

The caudal two-thirds of the medulla contains the rostral continuation of the central canal of the spinal cord and is, therefore, sometimes referred to as the 'closed' portion of the medulla. In passing rostrally, the central canal moves progressively more dorsally until, in the rostral medulla, it opens out into the fourth ventricle. This portion is sometimes referred to as the 'open' medulla. The floor of the fourth ventricle forms a shallow, rhomboid depression on the dorsal surface of the rostral medulla and the pons. The transition from medulla to pons is not clearly delineated on the dorsal surface of the brain stem but, approximately, the caudal third of the floor of the fourth ventricle constitutes the dorsal aspect of the rostral medulla, while the rostral two-thirds of the ventricular floor is made up of the dorsal aspect of the pons. The fourth ventricle is widest at the level of the pontomedullary junction where a **lateral recess** extends to the lateral margin of the brain stem. At this point the small **lateral aperture (foramen of Luschka)** provides passage for CSF within the fourth ventricle to reach the subarachnoid space surrounding the brain. The lateral walls of the rostral part of the fourth ventricle are made up of the **superior** and **inferior cerebellar peduncles**, connecting the brain stem with the cerebellum. In the rostral pons, the walls converge until, at the pontomesencephalic junction, the fourth ventricle becomes continuous with a small channel, the **cerebral aqueduct**, which passes throughout the length of the midbrain.

The dorsal aspect of the midbrain is marked by four paired elevations, the **superior** and **inferior colliculi**, which are parts of the visual and auditory

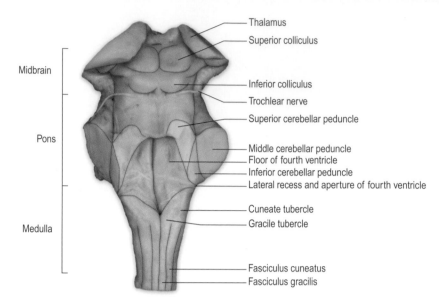

Figure 9.1 **Dorsal aspect of the brain stem.**

Figure 9.2 **Lateral aspect of the brain stem.**

systems, respectively. The **trochlear nerve** (IV cranial nerve) emerges immediately caudal to the inferior colliculus.

Ventral surface of the brain stem

On the ventral surface of the medulla, prominent longitudinal columns, the pyramids, run on either side of the ventral median fissure (Figs 9.3, 9.4). The pyramid gives its name to the underlying **pyramidal** or **corticospinal tract**, which consists of descending fibres originating from the ipsilateral cerebral cortex. In the caudal medulla, 75–90% of these fibres cross over in the **decussation of the pyramids** (Figs 9.3–9.5), partly obscuring the ventral median fissure as they do so, to form the lateral corticospinal tract of the spinal cord. Lateral to the pyramid lies an elongated elevation, the **olive**, within which lies the

inferior olivary nucleus. This has connections primarily with the cerebellum and is involved in the control of movement.

The transition from medulla to pons is clearly delineated on the ventral surface of the brain stem. The ventral part of the pons is dominated by a transverse system of fibres (the **transverse pontine fibres** or **pontocerebellar fibres**) that originate from cells in the ventral pons (**pontine nuclei**) and pass through the contralateral **middle cerebellar peduncle** to enter the cerebellar hemisphere. The pontine nuclei receive corticopontine fibres from the cerebral cortex (including the motor cortex) and constitute an important connection between cerebral and cerebellar cortices involved in the coordination of movement. The massive system of transverse pontine fibres obscures the underlying corticospinal tract.

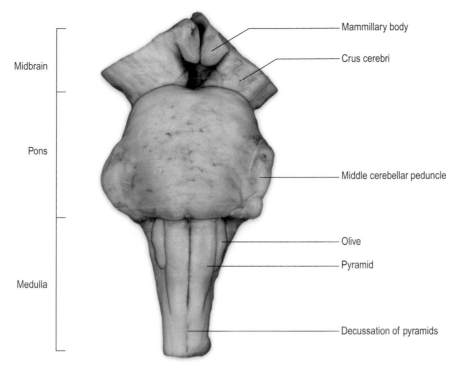

Figure 9.3 **Ventral aspect of the brain stem.**

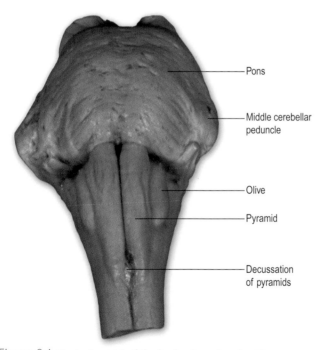

Figure 9.4 **Ventral aspect of the brain stem showing the decussation of the pyramids.**

The ventral surface of the midbrain consists, on either side, of a large column of descending fibres, the **crus cerebri** or **basis pedunculi**. In the midline, the two crura cerebri are separated by a depression called the interpeduncular fossa. The crus cerebri is continuous rostrally with the internal capsule of the cerebral hemisphere (Fig. 1.23) and consists of corticobulbar and corticospinal fibres that have left the cerebral hemisphere via the internal capsule on their way to the brain stem and spinal cord. They are primarily motor in function.

External features of the brain stem

- The brain stem consists of the medulla oblongata, pons and midbrain.
- On the dorsal aspect of the brain stem can be seen the dorsal columns, the floor of the fourth ventricle and the superior and inferior colliculi.
- The dorsal aspect of the rostral medulla and the pons form the floor of the fourth ventricle; the lateral and median apertures of the fourth ventricle permit the passage of CSF into the subarachnoid space. The cerebral aqueduct runs through the midbrain, beneath the colliculi.
- On the ventral aspect of the brain stem can be seen the pyramids, transverse pontine fibres and the crura cerebri.
- The inferior, middle and superior cerebellar peduncles connect the cerebellum to the medulla, pons and midbrain, respectively.

Internal structure of the brain stem

Caudal medulla

At the transition from spinal cord to medulla, the pattern of grey and white matter undergoes considerable rearrangement (Fig. 9.5). The ventral horn becomes much attenuated. The dorsal horn is replaced by the caudal part of the **trigeminal sensory nucleus (nucleus of the spinal tract of the trigeminal nerve)**. The trigeminal sensory nucleus is regarded as the brain stem homologue of the dorsal horn since it receives primary afferent fibres conveying general sensation from the head, which enter the brain stem in the trigeminal nerve. It is a large nucleus that extends the whole length of the brain stem and into the upper segments of the spinal cord. This latter, caudal part of the trigeminal nucleus is particularly associated with the modalities of pain and temperature. The trigeminal nerve

Fasciculus cuneatus

Nucleus cuneatus

Central grey

Spinocerebellar tracts

Pyramid

Fasciculus gracilis

Nucleus gracilis

Spinal tract of trigeminal

Nucleus of spinal tract of trigeminal

Decussation of pyramids

Figure 9.5 **Transverse section through the caudal medulla at the level of the decussation of the pyramids.** The sections shown in Figs 9.5–9.13 have been stained by the Weigert–Pal method. Areas rich in nerve fibres stain darkly, while areas rich in cell bodies are relatively pale.

Central grey

Fasciculus cuneatus

Nucleus cuneatus

Spinocerebellar tracts

Pyramid

Fasciculus gracilis

Nucleus gracilis

Spinal tract of trigeminal

Nucleus of spinal tract of trigeminal

Internal arcuate fibres

Medial lemniscus

Decussation of internal arcuate fibres

Figure 9.6 **Transverse section through the mid-medulla at the level of the great sensory decussation.**

attaches to the pons and, therefore, fibres that terminate in the parts of the trigeminal nucleus caudal to this level descend in a tract (**the spinal tract of the trigeminal**) which lies immediately superficial to the nucleus.

In the ventral medulla, the majority of fibres of the pyramid undergo decussation and then pass laterally, dorsally and caudally to form the lateral corticospinal tract.

Mid-medulla

On the ventral surface of the mid-medulla the pyramids are prominent, above their decussation. On the dorsal surface, the ascending fibres of the dorsal columns reach their termination in the gracile and cuneate nuclei, which appear beneath their respective tracts (Fig. 9.6). The dorsal columns consist of first-order sensory neurones; the cell bodies of these neurones lie in the dorsal root ganglia of spinal nerves and have central processes that ascended ipsilaterally through the cord and into the medulla. They terminate in the nuclei gracilis and cuneatus, upon the cell bodies of second-order neurones. The axons of the second-order neurones course ventrally and medially as **internal arcuate**

fibres, decussating in the midline. Thereafter, they turn rostrally forming a distinct tract, the **medial lemniscus**, which runs through the rostral medulla, the pons and midbrain to terminate upon third-order neurones in the ventral posterior nucleus of the thalamus.

Rostral medulla

Passing into the rostral medulla a number of new features appear, mostly related to the ventricular system and cerebellar connections. On the ventral surface of the medulla, the descending fibres of the pyramids remain conspicuous. Immediately dorsal to the medial aspect of the pyramid lie the ascending fibres of the medial lemniscus, on either side of the midline (Fig. 9.7). Dorsolateral to the pyramid and lateral to the medial lemniscus is the **inferior olivary nucleus**, lying within the prominence of the olive. The inferior olivary nucleus has roughly the form of a crenated bag with an opening, or hilum, facing medially, through which afferent and efferent fibres pass. The nucleus is concerned with the control of movement and receives afferents from the motor and sensory cortices of the

Figure 9.7 **Transverse section through the rostral medulla at the level of the inferior olivary nucleus.**

cerebral hemisphere and from the red nucleus of the midbrain. Its main efferent connection is to the cerebellum via the inferior cerebellar peduncle. Within the cerebellum, axons originating from the inferior olivary nucleus, known as climbing fibres, end in excitatory synapses in the dentate nucleus and upon Purkinje cells of the cerebellar cortex.

Dorsal to the inferior olivary nucleus and lateral to the medial lemniscus lie second-order sensory fibres ascending to the ventral posterior thalamus from the trigeminal nucleus (the **trigeminothalamic tract** or **trigeminal lemniscus**) and from the spinal cord (spinothalamic fibres, referred to in the brain stem as the **spinal lemniscus**).

The dorsal surface of the rostral medulla forms part of the floor of the fourth ventricle. Both immediately and deep beneath the floor of the ventricle lie a number of cranial nerve nuclei, some of which can be clearly identified in simply stained sections, others of which cannot. Immediately beneath the ventricular floor, just lateral to the midline, lies the **hypoglossal nucleus**, which contains motor neurones innervating the muscles of the tongue via the hypoglossal nerve. Lateral to the hypoglossal nucleus lies the **dorsal motor nucleus of the vagus**, containing preganglionic parasympathetic neurones that run in the vagus nerve. The most caudal aspect of the ventricular floor is known as the **area postrema**. At this point, the blood–brain barrier, which limits the passage of certain chemicals from the blood to the brain, is absent. This region is the central site of action of substances that cause vomiting (emetics). In the lateral part of the floor of the fourth ventricle are located the **vestibular nuclei**, which receive primary afferent fibres from the vestibular nerve. Ventromedial to the hypoglossal nucleus, close to the midline, is located the **medial longitudinal fasciculus**. This consists of both ascending and descending fibres and can be identified also in the pons and midbrain. Within the brain stem, it links the vestibular nuclei with the nuclei supplying the extraocular muscles (abducens, trochlear and oculomotor nuclei) and subserves the coordination of head and eye movements.

The dorsolateral part of the rostral medulla is dominated by the inferior cerebellar peduncle, or **restiform body**. This consists of fibres passing between the medulla and the cerebellum. Prominent among these are olivocerebellar fibres, connections between the vestibular nuclei and the

cerebellum, and the fibres of the dorsal spinocerebellar tract, conveying proprioceptive information from the limbs. On the dorsal and lateral aspects of the inferior cerebellar peduncle lie the dorsal and ventral **cochlear nuclei**, which receive afferent fibres from the cochlear nerve. Deep beneath the ventricular floor, just dorsal to the inferior olivary nucleus, is located the **nucleus ambiguus**. This sends motor fibres into the glossopharyngeal, vagus and accessory nerves and, thence, to the muscles of the pharynx and larynx.

Pons

The pons may be divided into a ventral, or basal, portion and a dorsal portion, also known as the **tegmentum**. The ventral portion is marked by numerous transversely oriented fascicles of pontocerebellar fibres that originate from scattered cell groups, the **pontine nuclei**, and pass into the contralateral side of the cerebellum through the massive middle cerebellar peduncle (**brachium pontis**) (Figs 9.8–9.10). Corticospinal fibres (which continue into the medullary pyramid) appear as small, separate bundles running longitudinally between the fascicles of transverse pontine fibres.

The ascending fibres of the medial lemniscus become separated from the pyramid and displaced dorsally, together with the spinal lemniscus and trigeminothalamic tract (trigeminal lemniscus), by intervening transverse pontocerebellar fibres. The medial lemniscus also rotates through 90° so that it lies almost horizontally, marking the boundary between ventral and tegmental portions of the pons. In the caudal pons (Fig. 9.8), an additional group of transversely running fibres is located ventral to the ascending lemniscal fibres but dorsal to the pontocerebellar fibres. This is the **trapezoid body**, which consists of acoustic fibres crossing the brain stem from the cochlear nuclei. They ascend into the midbrain as the **lateral lemniscus** and terminate in the inferior colliculus.

Beneath the floor of the fourth ventricle, in the pontine tegmentum, lie a number of cranial nerve nuclei. These include the **abducens nucleus** (innervating the lateral rectus muscle), the **facial motor nucleus** (innervating the muscles of facial expression) and the **trigeminal motor nucleus** (innervating the muscles of mastication), which each supply motor axons to their respective cranial nerves.

Cerebellum
Choroid plexus
Fourth ventricle
Medial longitudinal fasciculus
Medial lemniscus
Pontine nuclei
Corticospinal fibres

Dentate nucleus
Middle cerebellar peduncle
Abducens nucleus
Pontocerebellar fibres

Figure 9.8 **Transverse section through the caudal pons.**

Fourth ventricle
Medial longitudinal fasciculus
Medial lemniscus
Pontine nuclei
Corticospinal fibres

Superior cerebellar peduncle
Middle cerebellar peduncle
Reticular formation
Trigeminal nerve
Pontocerebellar fibres

Figure 9.9 **Transverse section through the mid-pons at the level of the trigeminal nerve.**

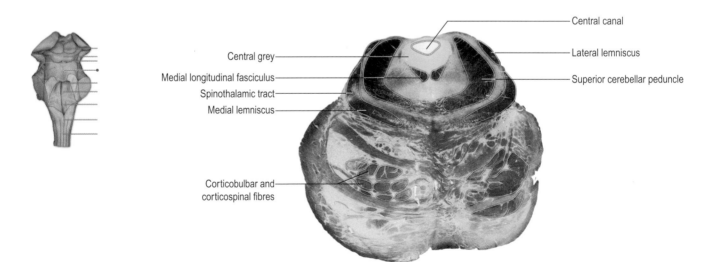

Central grey
Medial longitudinal fasciculus
Spinothalamic tract
Medial lemniscus
Corticobulbar and corticospinal fibres

Central canal
Lateral lemniscus
Superior cerebellar peduncle

Figure 9.10 **Transverse section through the rostral pons.**

Also the trigeminal sensory nucleus, already encountered in the medulla, reaches its maximum extent in the pons, adjacent to the origin of the trigeminal nerve.

In the rostral part of the pons (Fig. 9.10) the superior cerebellar peduncles form the lateral walls of the fourth ventricle, the thin superior medullary velum spanning between them to form its roof. The superior peduncle contains some cerebellar afferent fibres, such as the ventral spinocerebellar tract, which conveys proprioceptive information from the limbs. It consists mainly, however, of ascending cerebellar efferents concerned with the coordination of movement, that are destined for the red nucleus of the midbrain and the ventral lateral nucleus of the thalamus. The superior cerebellar peduncles converge towards the midline as they pass into the midbrain.

Midbrain

The midbrain is formally divided into dorsal and ventral portions at the level of the cerebral aqueduct. The dorsal portion is known as the **tectum**, which consists largely of the **inferior** and **superior colliculi (corpora quadrigemina)**. The ventral portion of the midbrain is known as the **tegmentum**. It is bounded ventrally by the massive fibre system of the crus cerebri. The term **cerebral peduncle** is sometimes used as a synonym for crus cerebri, but strictly speaking, the cerebral peduncle refers to the whole of the ventral midbrain, on either side, excluding the tectum.

In the caudal part of the midbrain, the inferior colliculus constitutes part of the **ascending acoustic (auditory) projection**. Ascending auditory fibres run in the lateral lemniscus, which terminates in the inferior colliculus. Efferent fibres from the colliculus terminate in the **medial geniculate nucleus** of the thalamus, which in turn projects to the auditory cortex of the temporal lobe.

The superior colliculus of the rostral midbrain is part of the visual system. Its main afferents are corticotectal fibres originating from the visual cortex of the occipital lobe and

from the frontal eye field of the frontal lobe. These inputs are concerned with controlling movements of the eyes, such as those occurring when a moving object is followed (smooth pursuit) or when the direction of the gaze is altered (saccadic eye movements). In addition, corticotectal fibres from the visual cortex are involved in the **accommodation reflex** (Ch. 10).

A small number of visual fibres running in the optic tract terminate just rostral to the superior colliculus, in the **pretectal nucleus**. This nucleus has connections with parasympathetic neurones controlling the smooth muscle of the eye and is part of the circuit mediating the **pupillary light reflex** (Ch. 10)

Ventral to the colliculi, the cerebral aqueduct runs the length of the midbrain. Surrounding the aqueduct is a pear-shaped arrangement of grey matter, the **periaqueductal (or central) grey**. In the ventral part of the periaqueductal grey, at the levels of the inferior and superior colliculi, respectively, lie the **trochlear and oculomotor nuclei**, which innervate the extraocular muscles controlling eye movements. Close to the nuclei runs the medial longitudinal fasciculus, which links them to the abducens nucleus in the pons and is important in the control of gaze.

At the level of the inferior colliculus (Figs 9.11, 9.12), the central portion of the tegmentum is dominated by the superior cerebellar peduncles (**brachium conjunctivum**).

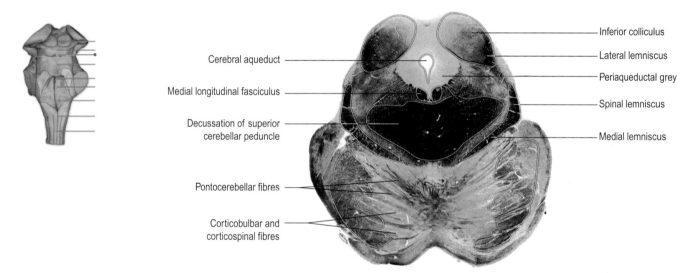

Cerebral aqueduct
Medial longitudinal fasciculus
Decussation of superior cerebellar peduncle
Pontocerebellar fibres
Corticobulbar and corticospinal fibres

Inferior colliculus
Lateral lemniscus
Periaqueductal grey
Spinal lemniscus
Medial lemniscus

Figure 9.11 **Transverse section through the brain stem at the level of the pontine–mesencephalic junction.**

Cerebral aqueduct
Periaqueductal grey
Spinal lemniscus
Medial longitudinal fasciculus
Medial lemniscus
Superior cerebellar peduncle
Decussation of superior cerebellar peduncle
Substantia nigra

Inferior colliculus
Lateral lemniscus
Trochlear nucleus
Temporopontine fibres
Corticobulbar and corticospinal fibres
Frontopontine fibres

Crus cerebri

Figure 9.12 **Transverse section through the caudal midbrain at the level of the inferior colliculus.**

Figure 9.13 **Transverse section through the rostral midbrain at the level of the superior colliculus.**

These fibres originate in the cerebellum, coursing ventromedially as they run into the midbrain. Beneath the inferior colliculus, the superior cerebellar peduncles decussate in the midline. Rostral to the decussation, at the level of the superior colliculus (Fig. 9.13), the central portion of the tegmentum is occupied by the **red nucleus**, in which some of the fibres of the superior cerebellar peduncle terminate. The red nucleus is involved in motor control. Its other major source of afferents is the motor cortex of the frontal lobe. Efferent fibres from the red nucleus cross in the ventral tegmental decussation and descend to the spinal cord in the **rubrospinal tract**. In addition, the red nucleus projects to the inferior olivary nucleus of the medulla, via the **central tegmental tract**.

The most ventral part of the midbrain tegmentum is occupied by the **substantia nigra**. A subdivision of this nucleus, known as the **pars compacta**, consists of pigmented, melanin-containing neurones that synthesise dopamine as their transmitter. These neurones project to the caudate nucleus and putamen of the basal ganglia in the forebrain (Ch. 14). Degeneration of the pars compacta of the substantia nigra is associated with Parkinson's disease. The other, non-pigmented, subdivision of the substantia nigra is called the **pars reticulata**. It is considered to be a functional homologue of the medial segment of the globus pallidus, which is also part of the basal ganglia.

Ventral to the substantia nigra lies the massive crus cerebri. This consists entirely of descending cortical efferent fibres that have left the cerebral hemisphere by traversing the internal capsule. Approximately the middle 50% of the crus consists of **corticobulbar** and **corticospinal fibres**. The corticobulbar fibres end predominantly in or near the motor cranial nerve nuclei of the brain stem. The corticospinal (pyramidal) fibres traverse the pons to enter the medullary pyramid and, thence, the corticospinal tracts.

On either side of the corticobulbar and corticospinal fibres, the crus cerebri contains corticopontine fibres that originate from widespread regions of the cerebral cortex and terminate in the pontine nuclei of the ventral pons. From the pontine nuclei connections are established with the cerebellum, via the middle cerebellar peduncle, that are involved in the coordination of movement.

Reticular formation

The reticular formation consists of a complex matrix of neurones that extends throughout the length of the brain stem. This is, in phylogenetic terms, a relatively old part of the brain stem and its neurones fulfil a number of important functions, some of which are necessary for survival. The reticular formation has widespread afferent and efferent connections with other parts of the CNS, which reflect its complex and multimodal functions. Some reticular neurones have long axons that ascend and descend for considerable distances within the brain stem, allowing profuse interaction with other neuronal systems. Within the reticular formation a number of individual nuclei are recognised. Some functions are subserved, however, by more dispersed networks that do not correspond exactly to anatomically identified nuclei. The latter applies to the so-called respiratory and cardiovascular centres. These consist of diffuse neuronal networks located within the medullary and caudal pontine reticular formation that control respiratory movements and cardiovascular function.

Internal structure of the brain stem

- Cranial nerves III–XII attach to the brain stem, their fibres either originating from, or terminating in, the cranial nerve nuclei.
- The reticular formation controls the level of consciousness, the cardiovascular system and the respiratory system.
- Ascending sensory systems pass through the brain stem en route to the thalamus. First-order proprioceptive fibres in the dorsal columns relay in the dorsal column nuclei. Second-order fibres decussate to form the medial lemniscus. Spinothalamic fibres form the spinal lemniscus. Second-order fibres originating in the trigeminal sensory nucleus constitute the trigeminothalamic tract (trigeminal lemniscus).
- Descending fibre systems end in the brain stem, pass through it and originate within it.
- Corticobulbar fibres terminate in the midbrain, pons and medulla. The corticospinal tract runs through the crus cerebri, the basal part of the pons and the medullary pyramid; 75–90% of fibres cross in the pyramidal decussation to form the lateral corticospinal tract.
- The reticular formation, red nucleus and vestibular nuclei give rise to descending fibres that pass to the spinal cord.

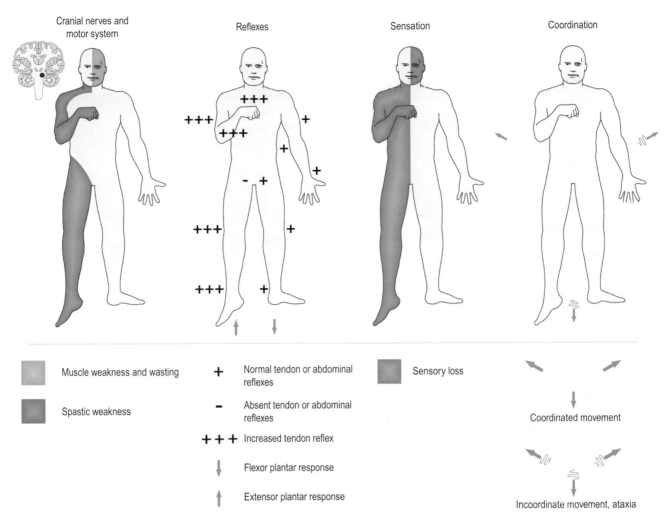

| Cranial nerves and motor system | Reflexes | Sensation | Coordination |

Muscle weakness and wasting	$+$	Normal tendon or abdominal reflexes		Sensory loss	
Spastic weakness	$-$	Absent tendon or abdominal reflexes			Coordinated movement
	$+++$	Increased tendon reflex			
	↓	Flexor plantar response			
	↑	Extensor plantar response			Incoordinate movement, ataxia

Figure 9.14 **Brain stem lesion.**

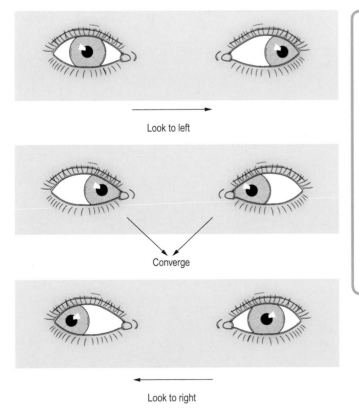

Look to left

Converge

Look to right

Figure 9.15 **Internuclear ophthalmoplegia.**

Brain stem lesions

A unilateral brain stem lesion caused by stroke, tumour or multiple sclerosis causes ipsilateral cranial nerve dysfunction, contralateral spastic hemiparesis, hyperreflexia and an extensor plantar response (upper motor neurone lesion), contralateral hemisensory loss and ipsilateral incoordination (Fig. 9.14). A bilateral lesion destroys the 'vital centres' for respiration and the circulation, leading to coma and death. Multiple sclerosis can affect eye movements through demyelination of the medial longitudinal fasciculus, which interferes with conjugate ocular deviation. Typically, on horizontal gaze, the abducting eye moves normally but the adducting eye fails to follow. Adduction is preserved on convergence. **Internuclear ophthalmoplegia** is the term used to describe this disorder (Fig. 9.15).

Descending **reticulospinal tracts** originate from the medullary and pontine reticular formation (Ch. 8). These predominantly influence muscle tone and posture. Some of the ascending fibres of the reticular formation constitute the **reticular activating system**. These neurones receive input, either directly or indirectly, from multiple sensory sources. Through the intermediary of thalamic nuclei, they cause activation of the cerebral cortex and heightened arousal.

The **raphé nuclei** are a group of midline nuclei that extend throughout the length of the brain stem. Many of the neurones of these nuclei are serotonergic, utilising serotonin (5-hydroxytryptamine, 5-HT) as their transmitter. Their axons are widely distributed throughout the CNS. In particular, ascending fibres to forebrain structures are involved in the neural mechanisms of sleep, and descending fibres to the spinal cord are involved in the modulation of nociceptive mechanisms.

The **locus coeruleus** is a group of pigmented neurones that lies in the brain stem tegmentum of the caudal midbrain and rostral pons. It is the principal noradrenergic cell group of the brain. It projects to many areas of the CNS. Ascending fibres project to the cerebellum, hypothalamus, thalamus, limbic structures and cerebral cortex. Descending fibres project widely throughout the brain stem and spinal cord. The locus coeruleus, like the raphé nuclei, has been implicated in the neural mechanisms regulating sleep, particularly REM (rapid eye movement) sleep.

Chapter 10
Cranial nerves and cranial nerve nuclei

There are twelve (XII), bilaterally paired, cranial nerves; these carry afferent and efferent fibres between the brain and peripheral structures, principally of the head and neck. The cranial nerves are individually named and numbered (Roman numerals) according to the rostrocaudal sequence in which they attach to the brain (Fig. 10.1 and Table 10.1):

I olfactory	VII facial
II optic	VIII vestibulocochlear
III oculomotor	IX glossopharyngeal
IV trochlear	X vagus
V trigeminal	XI accessory
VI abducens	XII hypoglossal

The first two cranial nerves attach directly to the forebrain, while the rest attach to the brain stem. The olfactory system is closely associated, both structurally and functionally, with parts of the forebrain collectively referred to as the limbic system; these, including cranial nerve I, are considered together in Chapter 16. The visual system and cranial nerve II are described in Chapter 15. Cranial nerves III–XII are associated with various nuclei within the brain stem, called the cranial nerve nuclei, which either receive cranial nerve afferents or contain the cell bodies of efferent neurones that have axons leaving the brain in cranial nerves. The locations of these nuclei are illustrated in Figure 10.2.

Cranial nerve nuclei

Afferent nuclei
Fibres carrying general sensory information (touch, pressure, pain, temperature) from the head enter the brain through the trigeminal nerve at the level of the pons and terminate in the **trigeminal sensory nucleus**. This is a large nucleus that runs the whole length of the brain stem and extends caudally into the cervical spinal cord. Fibres conveying the special senses of motion/positional sense and hearing run in the vestibulocochlear nerve. They terminate in the **vestibular** and **cochlear nuclei**, respectively, which are located in the medulla, in and near to the lateral part of the floor of the fourth ventricle (sometimes referred to as the vestibular area). Visceral afferents, including taste fibres, terminate in the **nucleus solitarius** of the medulla.

Efferent nuclei
On the basis of their embryological derivation, the efferent cranial nerve nuclei can be divided into three groups, each lying in a discontinuous longitudinal column.

Nuclei of the somatic efferent cell column
The somatic efferent cell column lies near to the midline and consists of the nuclei of the III, IV, VI and XII nerves. The **oculomotor nucleus** lies in the ventral apex of the periaqueductal grey of the midbrain at the level of the superior colliculus. Its efferent fibres run in the oculomotor nerve to innervate the levator palpebrae superioris and all of the extraocular muscles, except the superior oblique and lateral rectus. The **trochlear nucleus** also lies in the midbrain, at the ventral border of the periaqueductal grey, but at the level of the inferior colliculus. Fibres leave in the trochlear nerve to innervate the superior oblique muscle of the eye. The **abducens nucleus** is located in the caudal pons beneath the floor of the fourth ventricle. Its efferents run in the abducens nerve and they innervate the lateral rectus muscle. In the medulla lies the **hypoglossal nucleus**, which innervates the intrinsic and extrinsic muscles of the tongue via the hypoglossal nerve.

Nuclei of the branchiomotor cell column
The branchiomotor cell column innervates striated muscles derived from the branchial arches. In the tegmentum of the mid-pons is located the **trigeminal motor nucleus**, which supplies fibres to the trigeminal nerve and innervates the

Figure 10.1 **The base of the brain illustrating the locations of the cranial nerves.** The points of attachment are shown, except for the trochlear nerve, which arises from the dorsal aspect of the brain stem.

Table 10.1 **Cranial nerves**

Cranial nerve		Component fibres	Structures innervated	Functions
I	Olfactory	Sensory	Olfactory epithelium via olfactory bulb	Olfaction
II	Optic	Sensory	Retina	Vision
III	Oculomotor	Motor	Superior, inferior and medial recti; inferior oblique; levator palpebrae superioris	Movement of the eyeball; elevation of upper eyelid
		Parasympathetic	Sphincter pupillae and ciliary muscle of the eyeball, via ciliary ganglion	Pupillary constriction and accommodation
IV	Trochlear	Motor	Superior oblique muscle	Movement of the eyeball
V	Trigeminal	Sensory	Face, scalp, cornea, nasal and oral cavities, cranial dura mater	General sensation
		Motor	Muscles of mastication	Opening and closing the mouth
			Tensor tympani muscle	Tension on tympanic membrane
VI	Abducens	Motor	Lateral rectus muscle	Movement of the eyeball
VII	Facial	Sensory	Anterior two-thirds of tongue	Taste
		Motor	Muscles of facial expression	Facial movement
			Stapedius muscle	Tension on bones of middle ear
		Parasympathetic	Salivary and lacrimal glands via submandibular and pterygopalatine ganglia	Salivation and lacrimation
VIII	Vestibulocochlear	Sensory	Vestibular apparatus	Vestibular sensation (position and movement of head)
			Cochlea	Hearing
IX	Glossopharyngeal	Sensory	Pharynx, posterior third of tongue	General sensation and taste
			Eustachian tube, middle ear	General sensation
			Carotid body and carotid sinus	Chemo- and baroreception
		Motor	Stylopharyngeus muscle	Swallowing
		Parasympathetic	Parotid salivary gland via otic ganglion	Salivation
X	Vagus	Sensory	Pharynx, larynx, oesophagus, external ear	General sensation
			Aortic bodies, aortic arch	Chemo- and baroreception
			Thoracic and abdominal viscera	Visceral sensation
		Motor	Soft palate, pharynx, larynx, upper oesophagus	Speech, swallowing
		Parasympathetic	Thoracic and abdominal viscera	Control of cardiovascular system, respiratory and gastrointestinal tracts
XI	Accessory	Motor	Sternomastoid and trapezius muscles	Movement of head and shoulder
XII	Hypoglossal	Motor	Intrinsic and extrinsic muscles of the tongue	Movement of the tongue

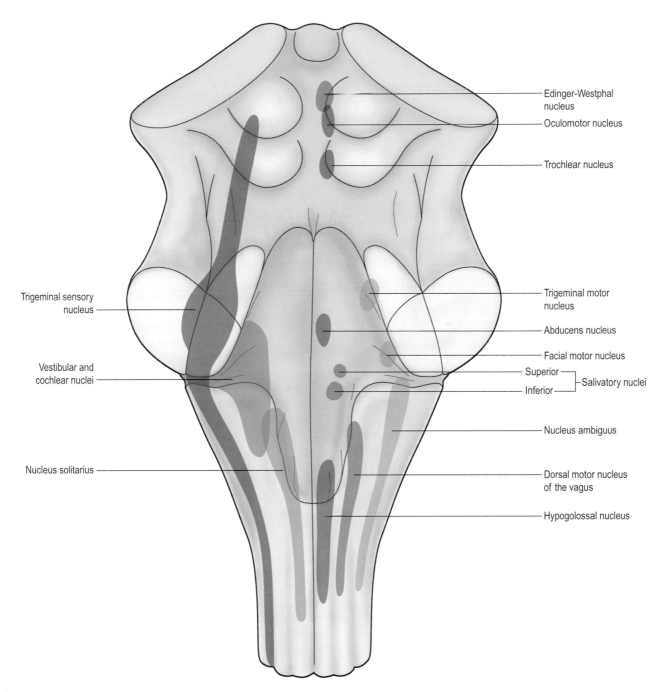

Figure 10.2 **The brain stem viewed from the dorsal aspect.** The diagram illustrates the locations of the afferent cranial nerve nuclei (left) and the efferent cranial nerve nuclei (right). On the right, nuclei shaded in the same colour share a common embryological origin.

muscles of mastication, tensor tympani, tensor veli palitini, mylohyoid and the anterior belly of the digastric muscle. In the caudal pontine tegmentum lies the **facial motor nucleus**. This innervates the muscles of facial expression and the stapedius muscle via the facial nerve. Within the medulla lies the **nucleus ambiguus**. This long nucleus sends motor fibres in the glossopharyngeal, vagus and cranial part of the accessory nerve to innervate the muscles of the pharynx and larynx.

Nuclei of the parasympathetic cell column

The parasympathetic cell column consists of preganglionic parasympathetic neurones that send axons into the III, VII, IX and X cranial nerves. The most rostral cell group constitutes the **Edinger–Westphal nucleus**, which lies in the midbrain periaqueductal grey matter adjacent to the oculomotor nucleus. Its axons leave in the oculomotor

nerve and pass to the ciliary ganglion in the orbit, from which postganglionic fibres innervate the sphincter pupillae and ciliary muscles within the eye.

In the pontine tegmentum lie two cell groups, the **superior** and **inferior salivatory nuclei**. The superior salivatory nucleus supplies preganglionic fibres to the facial nerve that terminate in the pterygopalatine and submandibular ganglia. Postganglionic fibres from the pterygopalatine ganglion innervate the lacrimal gland and the nasal and oral mucous membranes. Those from the submandibular ganglion innervate the submandibular and sublingual salivary glands. The inferior salivatory nucleus sends preganglionic fibres into the glossopharyngeal nerve. These terminate in the otic ganglion, which in turn sends postganglionic axons to the parotid salivary gland.

The largest preganglionic parasympathetic cell group lies in the medulla and constitutes the **dorsal motor nucleus**

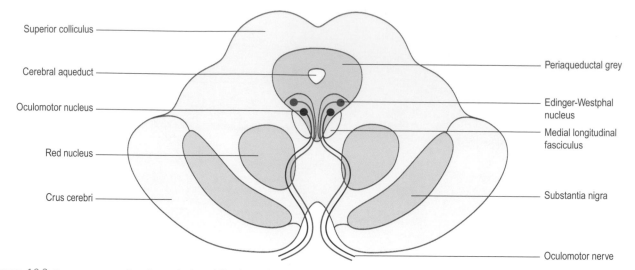

Figure 10.3 **Transverse section through the midbrain at the level of the superior colliculus.** The diagram shows the origin and course of oculomotor nerve fibres within the brain stem.

Figure 10.4 **Ventral aspect of the brain showing the points of attachment of cranial nerves I, II and III.**

of the vagus. Its rostral portion lies immediately beneath the floor of the fourth ventricle, lateral to the hypoglossal nucleus. Fibres leave in the vagus nerve and are widely distributed to thoracic and abdominal viscera.

Cranial nerves

III: Oculomotor nerve

The oculomotor nerve carries the majority of somatic motor neurones that innervate extraocular muscles and are responsible for moving the eye. It also contains preganglionic parasympathetic neurones that, via the intermediary of the ciliary ganglion, control the smooth muscle within the eye.

The motor neurones serving the extraocular muscles have their cell bodies in the **oculomotor nucleus**, which lies at the base of the periaqueductal grey of the midbrain at the level of the superior colliculus (Fig. 10.3). Preganglionic parasympathetic neurones arise from the nearby Edinger–

Westphal nucleus. Fibres from both sources course ventrally through the midbrain tegmentum, many of them traversing the red nucleus, to exit on the medial aspect of the crus cerebri, within the interpeduncular fossa (Fig. 10.4). The oculomotor nerve passes between the posterior cerebral and superior cerebellar arteries, then runs anteriorly, lying in the wall of the cavernous sinus (Fig. 7.11), before gaining access to the orbit through the superior orbital fissure. The oculomotor nerve supplies all of the extraocular muscles, with the exception of the superior oblique and lateral rectus and, thus, functions to elevate, depress and adduct the eyeball (Fig. 10.5). It also innervates the striated muscle of the levator palpebrae superioris, serving to elevate the upper eyelid. Preganglionic parasympathetic neurones terminate in the ciliary ganglion, located within the orbit, behind the eyeball. From here postganglionic neurones run in the **short ciliary nerves** to innervate the sphincter (constrictor) pupillae muscle of the iris and the ciliary muscle contained within the ciliary body.

Pupillary light reflex

The amount of light entering the eye is regulated by the size of the pupil. Illumination of the retina causes constriction of the pupil through contraction of the sphincter pupillae muscle of the iris, thus reducing the amount of light reaching the retina. This is known as the **direct light reflex** (Fig. 10.6). Even if only one retina is illuminated (e.g. during clinical examination) the pupils of both eyes constrict. The constriction of the pupil of the non-illuminated eye is called the **consensual light reflex**. The afferent limb of the light reflex consists of a small contingent of optic tract fibres that pass directly from the eye to the **pretectal area**, just rostral to the superior colliculus, rather than to the lateral geniculate nucleus of the thalamus where the majority of visual fibres terminate (see also Ch. 15). Neurones of the pretectal area project bilaterally to the Edinger–Westphal nuclei, from which efferent fibres leave in the oculomotor nerve.

Accommodation reflex

Fixation upon a nearby object, by convergence of the optic axes, involves concomitant contraction of the ciliary muscles to increase the convexity of the lens, thus focusing the image. It is also accompanied by pupillary constriction. The

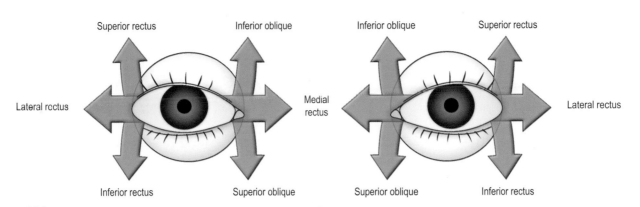

Figure 10.5 **Eye movements brought about by the extraocular muscles.**

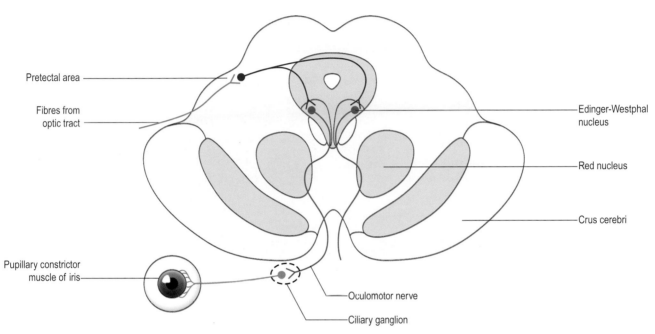

Figure 10.6 **Schematic representation of a transverse section through the most rostral part of the midbrain.** The diagram shows the pathways involved in the pupillary light reflex.

phenomenon involves the visual cortex, with corticobulbar fibres activating the parasympathetic neurones of the Edinger–Westphal nuclei bilaterally.

IV: Trochlear nerve

The trochlear nerve contains only somatic motor neurones. These arise in the **trochlear nucleus**, which lies in the ventral part of the midbrain periaqueductal grey, at the level of the inferior colliculus (Fig. 10.7). The efferent axons pass dorsally, around the periaqueductal grey, and decussate in the midline. The trochlear nerve emerges from the dorsal aspect of the brain stem (the only cranial nerve to do so) just caudal to the inferior colliculus (Fig. 10.8). The nerve courses round the cerebral peduncle to gain the ventral aspect of the brain (Fig. 10.9), passing between the posterior cerebral and superior cerebellar arteries, as does the oculomotor nerve. It then runs anteriorly, lying in the lateral wall of the cavernous sinus (Fig. 7.11) and enters the orbit through the superior orbital fissure. It supplies just one muscle, the **superior oblique**. The action of the superior oblique is complex. Depending upon the starting position of the eyeball it can act to depress, abduct or intort the eye. Importantly, with the eye adducted, the superior oblique depresses the visual axis. A lesion of the trochlear nerve

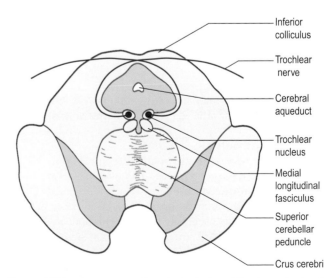

Figure 10.7 **Transverse section through the midbrain at the level of the inferior colliculus.** The diagram shows the location of the trochlear nucleus and the course of trochlear nerve fibres.

Figure 10.8 **Dorsal aspect of the brain stem, after removal of the cerebellum, showing the origin of the cranial nerve IV.**

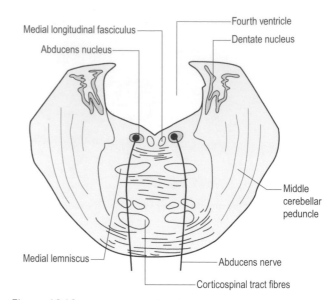

Figure 10.10 **Transverse section through the caudal pons.** The diagram shows the location of the abducens nucleus and the course of abducens nerve fibres.

Figure 10.9 **Ventral aspect of the brain showing cranial nerves III, IV and V.**

may, therefore, become manifest by diplopia on looking medially and downwards (e.g. when walking downstairs).

VI: Abducens nerve

The abducens nerve, like the trochlear, contains only somatic motor neurones. The cell bodies of origin are located in the **abducens nucleus**, which lies beneath the floor of the fourth ventricle in the caudal pons (Fig. 10.10). Efferent axons course ventrally through the pons and emerge from the ventral surface of the brain stem at the junction between the pons and the pyramid of the medulla (Fig. 10.11). The nerve then passes anteriorly, through the cavernous sinus (Fig. 7.11) and enters the orbit through the superior orbital fissure. The abducens supplies the lateral rectus muscle, which abducts the eye.

Lesions of cranial nerves III, IV and VI

A third cranial nerve palsy (Fig. 10.12) is caused by a lesion of the oculomotor nucleus within the midbrain or by compression of the peripheral course of cranial nerve III by an aneurysm or tumour. It leads to drooping of the eyelid (**ptosis**), dilation of the pupil that is unresponsive to light and accommodation, and an inability to move the eyeball upwards, downwards or inwards (adduction).

A sixth cranial nerve palsy (Fig. 10.13) is caused by a lesion of the abducens nucleus in the pons or by compression of the peripheral course of the nerve by an aneurysm or tumour. It leads to an inability to move the eye outwards (abduction).

Combined unilateral palsies of cranial nerves III, IV and VI occur from lesions along their peripheral course where the nerves run adjacent to each other, such as within the cavernous sinus, at the entrance to the orbit (superior orbital fissure syndrome) and within the orbit. There they are vulnerable to compression by tumours and aneurysms. The effects of such unilateral lesions are:

- ptosis
- dilation of the pupil that is unresponsive to light or accommodation
- paralysis of all eye movements (**ophthalmoplegia**) causing double vision (**diplopia**).

V: Trigeminal nerve

The trigeminal nerve has both sensory and motor components. It is the main sensory nerve for the head and, additionally, it innervates the muscles of mastication. It attaches to the brain stem as two adjacent roots (a large sensory and a smaller motor root) on the ventrolateral aspect of the pons, where this merges with the middle cerebellar peduncle (Figs 10.1, 10.9, 10.11).

Trochlear nerve — Pons — Trigeminal nerve — Facial nerve

Abducens nerve — Pyramid — Glossopharyngeal nerve — Vestibulocochlear nerve

Figure 10.11 **Ventral aspect of the brain showing the points of attachment of cranial nerves VI to IX.**

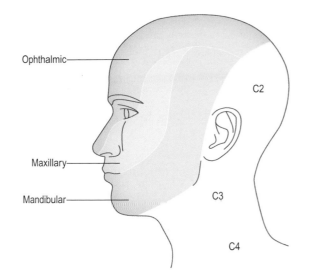

Ophthalmic

C2

Maxillary

Mandibular

C3

C4

Figure 10.14 **Superficial distribution of sensory fibres in the three divisions of the trigeminal nerve.**

(A)

(B)

Figure 10.12 **Right oculomotor (III) nerve palsy.** The upper part of the diagram shows ptosis on the right. The lower part shows that, with elevation of the eyelid, the eyeball can be seen to be abducted and the pupil dilated.

Figure 10.13 **Left abducens (VI) nerve palsy.** On looking in the direction of the arrow, the left eye fails to abduct.

The sensory fibres of the trigeminal nerve are primary sensory neurones with peripheral processes distributed via the ophthalmic, maxillary and mandibular divisions of the trigeminal to numerous structures of the head (Fig. 10.14). Sensations of touch, pressure, pain and temperature are relayed from the face and scalp, the cornea, the nasal and oral cavities, including the teeth and gums and the paranasal sinuses. The trigeminal nerve also innervates the intracranial dura mater and intracranial arteries. In addition,

proprioceptive fibres are carried from the muscles of mastication and the temporomandibular joint. The cell bodies of afferents in the trigeminal nerve, with the exception of those conveying proprioception, are located in the **trigeminal (or semilunar) ganglion**, located at the convergence of the ophthalmic, maxillary and mandibular nerves. The central processes of these cells terminate in the **trigeminal sensory nucleus** (Fig. 10.15).

The trigeminal sensory nucleus is a large nucleus that extends throughout the length of the brain stem and into the upper cervical spinal cord. It is considered to consist of three subnuclei. The **chief (or principal) sensory nucleus** lies in the pontine tegmentum close to the entry of the trigeminal nerve. The **mesencephalic nucleus** extends rostrally into the midbrain. The **spinal nucleus (or nucleus of the spinal tract of the trigeminal)** extends caudally through the medulla and into the cord, where it becomes continuous with the substantia gelatinosa, of which it is considered to be the brain stem homologue.

There is a segregated distribution of afferent fibre termination in the trigeminal nucleus, depending upon the modality. Fibres conveying touch and pressure terminate in the principal nucleus. Those carrying pain and temperature end in the spinal nucleus, reaching their termination by descending in the **spinal tract of the trigeminal**, a fascicle of fibres lying immediately superficial to the nucleus (Figs 9.5, 9.6). In the upper cervical cord, the spinal tract of the trigeminal becomes continuous with Lissauer's tract, which carries functionally homologous afferents of spinal nerve origin prior to their termination in the dorsal horn. Proprioceptive afferents from the muscles of mastication and the temporomandibular joint have their cell bodies not in the trigeminal ganglion, as might be expected, but in the mesencephalic nucleus of the trigeminal. They are the only primary afferents to have their cell bodies located within the CNS. Axons arising from second-order neurones in the trigeminal nucleus decussate to form the contralateral **trigeminothalamic tract (trigeminal lemniscus)**. This terminates in the contralateral ventral posterior nucleus of the thalamus, which in turn sends fibres to the sensory cortex of the parietal lobe. In addition, the trigeminal nucleus sends fibres to the cerebellum and also establishes reflex connections with certain motor cell groups of the

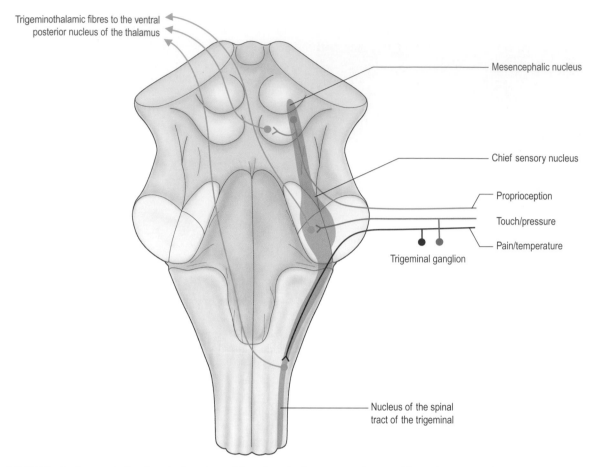

Figure 10.15 **The brain stem indicating the location of the trigeminal sensory nucleus and its major connections.**

brain stem. Prominent among these is the facial nucleus, through which are mediated facial grimacing and eye closure (corneal reflex) in response to noxious stimulation in the territory served by the trigeminal nerve.

> ### Lesions of the trigeminal nerve
> **Herpes zoster** infection of the sensory roots of the trigeminal nerve (**shingles**) leads to pain and the eruption of vesicles localised to the dermatome supplied by one or other of the ophthalmic, maxillary and mandibular branches of the trigeminal nerve.
>
> In **syringobulbia**, central cavitation of the medulla caudal to the fourth ventricle leads to preferential compressive destruction of decussating trigeminothalamic fibres, causing selective loss of pain and temperature sensibility (dissociated sensory loss) in the face (c.f. syringomyelia, p. 79).

The motor axons of the trigeminal nerve arise from cells in the trigeminal motor nucleus, which lies in the pontine tegmentum medial to the principal sensory nucleus (Fig. 10.2). Axons leave the pons in the motor root of the trigeminal and then join the mandibular division of the nerve. They innervate various muscles, the most significant of which are the muscles of mastication (masseter and temporalis, which close the jaw, and the lateral and medial pterygoids, which open the jaw). Trigeminal motor neurones also innervate tensor tympani within the middle ear, tensor veli palatini, mylohyoid and the anterior belly of digastric.

VII: Facial nerve

The facial nerve contains sensory, motor and parasympathetic components (Fig. 10.16). It joins the brain stem at the ventrolateral aspect of the caudal pons (Fig. 10.11), near the pontomedullary junction, in a region known as the **cerebellopontine angle**. The nerve consists of two roots, the more lateral (sometimes called the nervus intermedius) containing sensory and parasympathetic fibres, the more medial root being composed of motor axons.

The sensory fibres of the facial nerve supply taste sensation from the anterior two-thirds of the tongue, the floor of the mouth and palate, and also cutaneous sensation from part of the external ear. The cell bodies of primary afferent neurones lie in the **geniculate ganglion** within the facial canal of the petrous temporal bone. The central processes of taste fibres terminate in the rostral part of the nucleus solitarius of the medulla. Ascending fibres from the nucleus solitarius project to the ventral posterior nucleus of the thalamus, which in turn sends fibres to the sensory cortex of the parietal lobe. Afferent facial nerve fibres that carry cutaneous sensation terminate in the trigeminal nucleus.

Motor fibres of the facial nerve originate in the facial motor nucleus of the caudal pontine tegmentum (Fig. 10.17). The axons initially pass dorsally, looping over the abducens nucleus beneath the floor of the fourth ventricle, before leaving the brain stem in the motor root of the facial nerve. Motor fibres are distributed to the muscles of facial expression, platysma, stylohyoid, the posterior belly of the digastric muscle and the stapedius muscle of the middle ear.

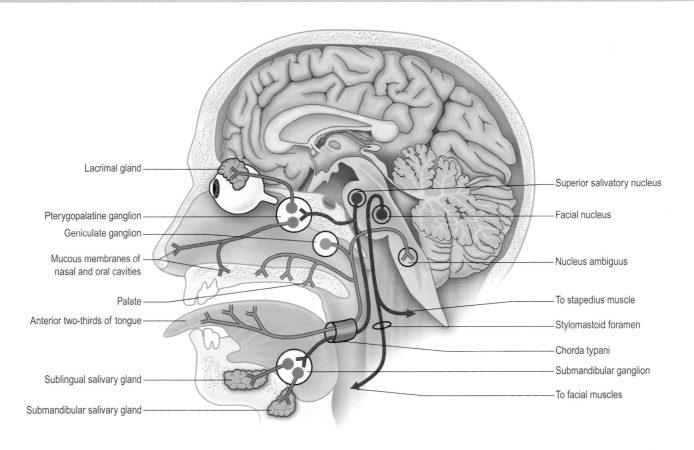

Figure 10.16 **Component fibres of the facial nerve and their peripheral distribution.** (Red, motor; blue, sensory; purple/orange, parasympathetic.)

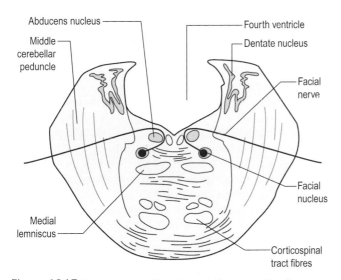

Figure 10.17 **Transverse section through the pons.** The diagram shows the origin and course of the motor fibres of the facial nerve.

The facial motor nucleus receives afferents from other brain stem areas for the mediation of certain reflexes and also from the cerebral cortex. Reflex connections are established that mediate protective eye closure in response to visual stimuli or tactile stimulation of the cornea (**corneal reflex**) through fibres from the superior colliculus and the trigeminal sensory nucleus, respectively. In addition, fibres from the superior olivary nucleus, a part of the central auditory pathway, subserve reflex contraction of the stapedius muscle in response to loud noise.

Corticobulbar fibres from motor cortical areas innervate the facial motor nucleus. Those that control motor neurones supplying the muscles of the upper face (frontalis, orbicularis oculi) are distributed bilaterally. Those that control the motor neurones supplying the muscles of the lower face are entirely crossed. Unilateral upper motor neurone lesions, therefore, give rise to paralysis of the lower facial muscles.

Preganglionic parasympathetic fibres of the facial nerve originate in the superior salivatory nucleus of the pons. Fibres leave the brain stem in the sensory root of the facial nerve (nervus intermedius). From here they pass to parasympathetic ganglia, namely the submandibular and pterygopalatine ganglia, where they synapse with postganglionic neurones. Postganglionic fibres from the submandibular ganglion innervate the submandibular and sublingual salivary glands. Those from the pterygopalatine ganglion innervate the lacrimal gland and the nasal and oral mucous membranes.

Bell's palsy

Bell's palsy represents an acute unilateral inflammatory lesion of the facial nerve within its course through the skull. Pain is experienced around the ear and there is paralysis of the facial muscles unilaterally with failure to close the eye, an absent corneal reflex, hyperacusis on the affected side and loss of taste sensation on the anterior two-thirds of the tongue. When the herpes zoster virus is the inflammatory agent, a vesicular rash is apparent in the external auditory canal and the mucous membrane of the oropharynx (**Ramsay Hunt syndrome**).

VIII: Vestibulocochlear nerve

The vestibulocochlear nerve is a sensory nerve that conveys impulses from the inner ear. It has two component parts: the **vestibular nerve**, which carries information related to position and movement of the head, and the **cochlear nerve**, which carries auditory information. Both divisions contain the axons of first-order sensory neurones, the dendrites of which make contact with hair cells of either the vestibular or auditory apparatus of the inner ear. Both divisions pass together through the internal auditory meatus (which also contains the facial nerve) and attach to the brain stem at the junction of the medulla and pons (Fig. 10.11), in the region known as the cerebellopontine angle.

The vestibular nerve

The vestibular nerve fibres make dendritic contact with **hair cells** of the vestibular portions of the membranous labyrinth; their cell bodies are located in the vestibular ganglion within the internal auditory meatus. The central processes of vestibular fibres mostly end in the **vestibular nuclei** of the rostral medulla. There are four such nuclei (superior, inferior, medial and lateral vestibular nuclei) located close together beneath the lateral part of the floor of the fourth ventricle.

The vestibular nuclei establish contact with a number of other regions for the control of posture, maintenance of equilibrium, coordination of head and eye movements, and the conscious awareness of vestibular stimulation. Fibres from the **lateral vestibular (Deiters')** nucleus descend ipsilaterally in the lateral vestibulospinal tract. The vestibular nuclei also contribute fibres to the **medial longitudinal fasciculus**. This extends throughout the brain stem and into the spinal cord; its descending component is also known as the medial vestibulospinal tract. Vestibulospinal fibres influence the activity of spinal motor neurones concerned with the control of body posture and balance. The ascending part of the medial longitudinal fasciculus establishes connections with the nuclei of the abducens, trochlear and oculomotor nerves for the coordination of head and eye movements. Some efferent fibres from the vestibular nuclei pass through the inferior cerebellar peduncle to the flocculonodular lobe of the cerebellum, which is concerned with the control of equilibrium. Other fibres ascend to the contralateral thalamus (ventral posterior nucleus), which in turn projects to the cerebral cortex. The cortical region responsible for conscious awareness of vestibular sensation is uncertain but is probably adjacent to the 'head' area of the sensory cortex in the parietal lobe or adjacent to the auditory cortex in the temporal lobe.

The cochlear nerve

The cochlear nerve fibres make dendritic contact with hair cells of the **organ of Corti** within the cochlear duct of the inner ear. The cell bodies of these fibres lie within the cochlea and are collectively called the spiral ganglion. The cochlear nerve joins the brain stem at the level of the rostral medulla. Its fibres bifurcate and end in the **dorsal** and **ventral cochlear nuclei**, which lie close to the inferior cerebellar peduncle. From here, the ascending auditory pathway to the thalamus and cerebral cortex (Fig. 10.18) is somewhat more complicated and variable than that for the general senses.

There are several locations between the medulla and thalamus where axons may synapse and not all fibres in the pathway behave in the same manner. From the cochlear nuclei, second-order neurones ascend into the pons, some of them crossing to the other side of the pontine tegmentum as the **trapezoid body**. At this level, some fibres may terminate in the **superior olivary nucleus**. This nucleus is the site of origin of olivocochlear fibres, which leave the brain stem in the vestibulocochlear nerve and end in the organ of Corti. They have an inhibitory function and serve to modulate transmission of auditory information to the cochlear nerve. From the superior olivary nuclei, ascending fibres comprise the **lateral lemniscus**, which runs through the pontine tegmentum to end in the **inferior colliculus** of the midbrain. Some axons within the lateral lemniscus terminate in a small pontine nucleus called the nucleus of the lateral lemniscus. The superior olivary nucleus and the nucleus of the lateral lemniscus are thought to establish reflex connections with motor neurones of the trigeminal and facial motor nuclei, mediating contraction of the tensor tympani and stapedius muscles in response to loud noise. The inferior colliculus, in turn, sends axons to the **medial geniculate nucleus** of the thalamus. The final step in the ascending auditory pathway consists of axons that originate in the medial geniculate nucleus and pass through the internal capsule to the **primary auditory cortex** of the temporal lobe. This is located predominantly in **Heschl's gyri** (Fig. 13.17), which are situated on the dorsal surface of the **superior temporal gyrus** and, therefore, are largely hidden within the lateral fissure. Throughout the ascending auditory projection, there exists a so-called 'tonotopical' representation of the cochlea, which is analogous to the 'somatotopic' organisation of the pathways for general sensation. Within the brain stem, some ascending fibres decussate while others do not. The representation of the cochlea is, therefore, bilateral at all levels rostral to the cochlear nuclei. For this reason, unilateral lesions of the ascending auditory pathway do not cause monaural deafness but, rather, are manifest as a loss of auditory acuity and an inability to localise the directional origin of sounds.

The region of the temporal lobe surrounding the primary auditory cortex is known as the **auditory association cortex** or **Wernicke's area**. It is here that auditory information is interpreted and given contextual significance. Wernicke's area is important in the processing of language by the brain (Ch. 13).

Acoustic neuroma

An acoustic neuroma is a benign tumour of the eighth cranial nerve which leads to compression of the nerve and adjacent structures in the **cerebellopontine angle**. Attacks of dizziness accompanied by profound deafness occur; with expansion of the tumour, ataxia and paralysis of the cranial nerves (especially V–VII) and the limbs follow. Unilateral and bilateral acoustic neuromas occur in the inherited disease **neurofibromatosis**, in which tumours of the peripheral nerves and skin (neurilemmoma and neurofibroma) can cause cosmetic blemish and deformity.

Figure 10.18 **Principal ascending connections of the auditory component of the vestibulocochlear nerve.**

IX: Glossopharyngeal nerve

The glossopharyngeal nerve is principally a sensory nerve, although it also contains preganglionic parasympathetic fibres and a few motor fibres. It attaches to the brain stem as a linear series of small rootlets, lateral to the olive in the rostral medulla (Figs 10.11, 10.19).

The afferent fibres of the glossopharyngeal nerve convey information from:

- receptors for general sensation in the pharynx, the posterior third of the tongue, Eustachian tube and middle ear
- taste buds of the pharynx and the posterior third of the tongue
- chemoreceptors in the carotid body and baroreceptors in the carotid sinus.

Figure 10.19 **Ventral aspect of the brain stem showing the points of attachment of cranial nerves VIII–XII.**

Within the brain stem, afferent fibres for general sensation end in the trigeminal sensory nucleus. Fibres carrying touch information from the pharynx and back of the tongue are important for mediating the **gag reflex**, through connections with the nucleus ambiguus and the hypoglossal nucleus. Visceral and taste fibres of the glossopharyngeal nerve terminate in the nucleus solitarius of the medulla.

The motor component of the glossopharyngeal nerve is very small. It arises from cells in the rostral part of the nucleus ambiguus of the medulla and innervates just one muscle, the stylopharyngeus, which is involved in swallowing.

Preganglionic parasympathetic fibres in the glossopharyngeal nerve originate in the inferior salivatory nucleus of the rostral medulla. These synapse with postganglionic neurones in the otic ganglion, which in turn innervate the parotid salivary gland.

X: Vagus nerve

Rootlets of the vagus nerve attach to the lateral aspect of the medulla immediately caudal to the glossopharyngeal nerve (Fig. 10.19). The vagus contains afferent, motor and parasympathetic fibres.

The afferent fibres of the vagus convey information from:

■ receptors for general sensation in the pharynx, larynx, oesophagus, tympanic membrane, external auditory meatus and part of the concha of the external ear

■ chemoreceptors in the aortic bodies and baroreceptors in the aortic arch

■ receptors widely distributed throughout the thoracic and abdominal viscera.

Within the brain stem, receptors for general sensation end in the trigeminal sensory nucleus, while visceral afferents end in the nucleus solitarius.

The motor fibres of the vagus (Fig. 10.20) arise from the nucleus ambiguus of the medulla. They innervate the muscles of the soft palate, pharynx, larynx and upper part of the oesophagus. The nucleus ambiguus is, therefore, crucially important in the control of speech and swallowing. By convention, the most caudal efferents from the nucleus ambiguus are regarded as leaving the brain stem in the cranial roots of the accessory nerve, but these transfer to the vagus nerve proper at the level of the jugular foramen (Fig. 10.20).

The parasympathetic fibres of the vagus nerve originate from the dorsal motor nucleus of the vagus, which lies in the medulla immediately beneath the floor of the fourth ventricle. They are distributed widely throughout the cardiovascular, respiratory and gastrointestinal systems.

XI: Accessory nerve

The accessory nerve is purely motor in function. It consists of two parts: cranial and spinal. The cranial part emerges from the lateral aspect of the medulla as a linear series of rootlets that lie immediately caudal to the rootlets of the

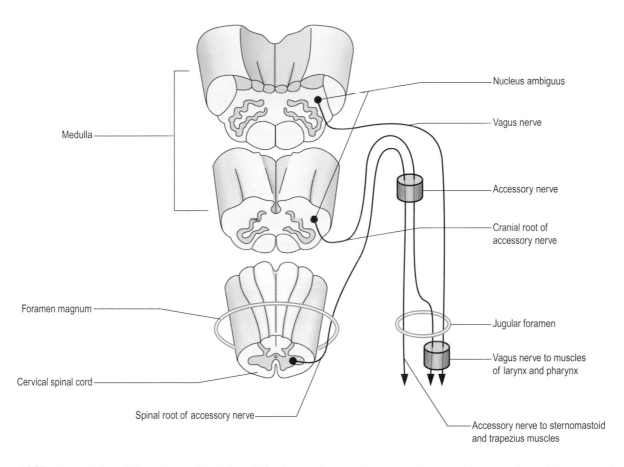

Figure 10.20 **The caudal medulla and rostral spinal cord.** The diagram illustrates the origin and course of the motor fibres of the vagus and accessory nerves.

vagus nerve (Figs 10.19, 10.20). The cranial root of the accessory nerve carries fibres that have their origin in the caudal part of the nucleus ambiguus of the medulla. At the level of the jugular foramen these fibres join the vagus nerve and are distributed with it to the muscles of the soft palate, pharynx and larynx.

The spinal root of the accessory nerve arises from motor neurones located in the ventral horn of the spinal grey matter at levels C1–C5 (Fig. 10.20). The axons leave the cord not through the ventral roots of spinal nerves but via a series of rootlets that emerge from the lateral aspect of the cord midway between the dorsal and ventral roots. These rootlets course rostrally, coalescing as they do so, and enter the cranial cavity through the foramen magnum. At the side of the medulla, the spinal root of the accessory nerve briefly joins the cranial root, but the component fibres separate once again as the nerve leaves the cranial cavity through the jugular foramen. Here the fibres of the cranial root of the accessory, which are derived from the nucleus ambiguus, join the vagus and are distributed with it. The fibres of the spinal root pass to the sternomastoid and trapezius muscles, which serve to move the head and shoulders.

XII: Hypoglossal nerve

The hypoglossal nerve is purely motor in function. It innervates both the extrinsic and intrinsic muscles of the tongue and, therefore, serves both to move the tongue and to change its shape. The axons originate in the hypoglossal nucleus, which lies immediately beneath the floor of the fourth ventricle, near the midline (Fig. 10.21). Axons course

ventrally through the medulla and emerge from its ventrolateral aspect as a linear series of rootlets located between the pyramid and the olive (Fig. 10.19). The hypoglossal nucleus receives afferents from the nucleus solitarius and the trigeminal sensory nucleus. These are involved in the control of the reflex movements of chewing, sucking and swallowing. It also receives corticobulbar fibres from the contralateral motor cortex, which subserve voluntary movements of the tongue such as occur in speech.

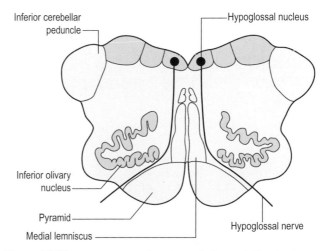

Figure 10.21 **Transverse section through the medulla.** The diagram shows the origin and course of the fibres of the hypoglossal nerve.

Motor neurone disease and lesions of cranial nerves IX–XII

Motor neurone disease is a chronic degenerative disorder seen in those aged over 50 years. The corticobulbar tracts projecting to the nucleus ambiguus and hypoglossal nucleus degenerate, leading to dysphonia (difficulty in phonation), dysphagia (difficulty in swallowing), dysarthria (difficulty in articulation) and weakness and spasticity of the tongue (**pseudobulbar palsy**). There is also degeneration of the nucleus ambiguus and hypoglossal nuclei themselves, leading to dysphonia, dysphagia, dysarthria and weakness, wasting and fasciculation of the tongue (**bulbar palsy**).

The IX, X, XI and XII nerves can be damaged by compression in their peripheral course as they exit the cranium via the foramina of the skull base. Tumours in this area lead to dysphonia and depression of the gag reflex, together with unilateral wasting of the sternomastoid and trapezius muscles (**jugular foramen syndrome**) and unilateral weakness, wasting and fasciculation of the tongue.

Chapter 11
Cerebellum

The cerebellum is the largest part of the hindbrain. It originates from the dorsal aspect of the brain stem and overlies the fourth ventricle. The cerebellum is connected to the brain stem by three stout pairs of fibre bundles, called the **inferior**, **middle** and **superior cerebellar peduncles** (Fig. 11.1); these join the cerebellum to the medulla, pons and midbrain, respectively. The functions of the cerebellum are entirely motor and it operates at an unconscious level. It controls the maintenance of equilibrium (balance), influences posture and muscle tone, and coordinates movement.

External features of the cerebellum

The cerebellum consists of two laterally located **hemispheres**, joined in the midline by the **vermis** (Figs 11.2–11.4). The superior surface of the cerebellum lies beneath the tentorium cerebelli and the superior vermis is raised, forming a midline ridge. Conversely, the inferior vermis lies in a deep groove between the hemispheres. The surface of the cerebellum is highly convoluted, the folds, or **folia**, being oriented approximately transversely. Between the folia lie fissures of varying depths. Some of these fissures are landmarks that are used to divide the cerebellum anatomically into three lobes (Figs 11.2–11.5). On the superior surface, the deep **primary fissure**

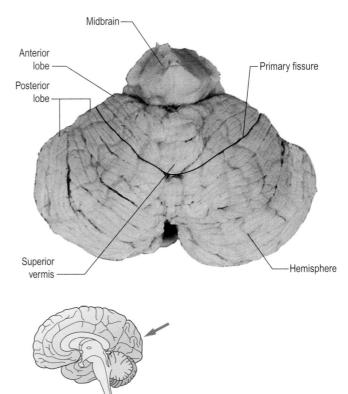

Figure 11.2 **Superior surface of the cerebellum.**

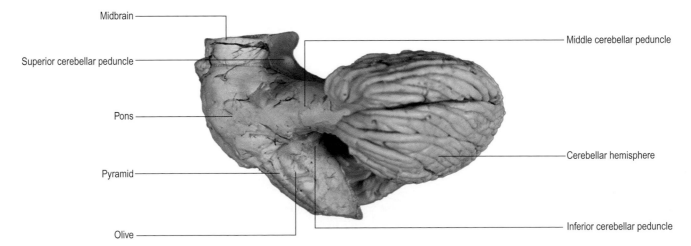

Figure 11.1 **Lateral aspect of the brain stem and cerebellum, showing the cerebellar peduncles.** Parts of the anterior, posterior and flocculonodular lobes have been removed to display the peduncles more clearly.

Figure 11.3 **Posterior aspect of the cerebellum.**

Figure 11.4 **Anteroinferior aspect of the cerebellum.**

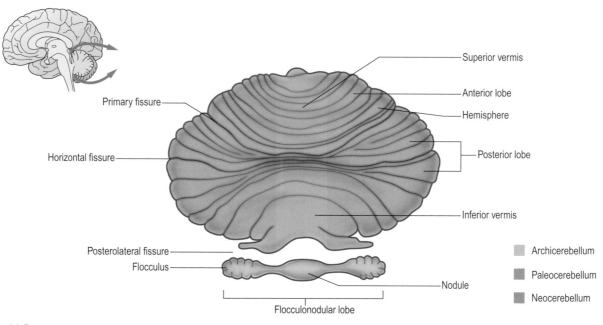

Figure 11.5 **Schematic representation of the cerebellum in which the peduncles have been cut and the surface flattened out.** The relationships between the anatomical and functional divisions of the cerebellum are shown.

External features of the cerebellum

- The cerebellum controls the maintenance of equilibrium, posture and muscle tone and it coordinates movement. It operates at an unconscious level.
- The cerebellum is connected to the medulla, pons and midbrain by the inferior, middle and superior cerebellar peduncles, respectively.
- The cerebellum consists of a midline vermis and two laterally located hemispheres.
- Anatomically, the cerebellum is divided into anterior, posterior and flocculonodular lobes.

separates the relatively small **anterior lobe** from the much larger **posterior lobe**. On the underside, the conspicuous **posterolateral fissure** demarcates the location of small regions of the hemisphere (the **flocculus**) and vermis (the **nodule**), which together form the **flocculonodular lobe**.

Internal structure of the cerebellum

The cerebellum basically consists of an outer layer of grey matter, the **cerebellar cortex**, and an inner core of white matter. The white matter is made up largely of afferent and efferent fibres that run to and from the cortex and towards which it extends irregular, branch-like projections, referred to in older literature as the arbor vitae (Figs 11.6, 11.7). Buried deep within the white matter are four pairs of **cerebellar nuclei** (Figs 11.6, 11.8), which have important connections with the cerebellar cortex and with certain nuclei of the brain stem and thalamus.

Cerebellar cortex

The cerebellar cortex is highly convoluted, forming numerous transversely oriented folia. Within the cortex lie the cell bodies, dendrites and synaptic connections of the vast majority of cerebellar neurones. The cellular organisation of the cortex is the same in all regions (Fig. 11.9). It is divided histologically into three layers:

1. The outer, fibre-rich, **molecular layer**
2. The intermediate, **Purkinje cell layer**

3. The inner **granular layer**, which is dominated by the **granule cell**.

Afferent projections to the cerebellum arise principally from the spinal cord (spinocerebellar fibres), inferior olivary nucleus (olivocerebellar fibres), vestibular nuclei (vestibulocerebellar fibres) and pons (pontocerebellar fibres). Afferent axons mostly terminate in the cerebellar cortex, where they are excitatory to cortical neurones. Fibres enter the cerebellum through one of the cerebellar peduncles and proceed to the cortex as either **mossy fibres** or **climbing fibres**, depending upon their origin (Fig. 11.10). All afferents originating elsewhere than the inferior olivary nucleus end as mossy fibres. Mossy fibres branch to supply several folia and end in the granular layer, in synaptic contact with granule cells. The axons of granule cells pass towards the surface of the cortex and enter the molecular layer. Here they bifurcate to produce two **parallel fibres** that are oriented along the long axis of the folium.

The Purkinje cell layer consists of a unicellular layer of the somata of Purkinje neurones. The profuse dendritic arborisations of these cells (see Fig. 2.1B) extend towards the surface of the cortex, into the molecular layer (Fig. 11.10). The arborisations are flattened and oriented at right angles to the long axis of the folium. They are, therefore, traversed by numerous parallel fibres, from which they receive excitatory synaptic input. Inhibitory modulation of intracortical circuitry is provided by numerous other neurones known as Golgi, basket and stellate cells. The axons of Purkinje cells are the only axons to leave the cerebellar cortex. Most of these fibres do not leave the cerebellum entirely but end in the deep cerebellar nuclei. The other type of afferent fibre entering the cerebellar cortex, the climbing fibre, originates from the inferior olivary nucleus of the medulla. These fibres provide relatively discrete excitatory input to Purkinje cells. At the same time, axon collaterals of climbing fibres excite the neurones of the deep cerebellar nuclei. Purkinje cells utilise GABA as their neurotransmitter, which means that the output of the whole of the cerebellar cortex is mediated through the inhibition of cells in the cerebellar nuclei.

Cerebellar nuclei

Deep within the cerebellar white matter, above the roof of the fourth ventricle, lie four pairs of nuclei. From medial to lateral, they are known as:

Dentate nucleus — White matter

Pons — Cerebellar cortex

Figure 11.6 **Parasagittal section through the cerebellum.** Mulligan's stain.

Cerebral hemisphere —

Dentate nucleus —

Cerebellar vermis —

— Cerebellar white matter

— Cerebellar hemisphere

— Medulla

Figure 11.7 **Coronal section of the brain at the level of the dentate nucleus;** myelin stain. (Section courtesy of the National Museum of Health and Medicine, Armed Forces Institute of Pathology, Washington, DC, USA.)

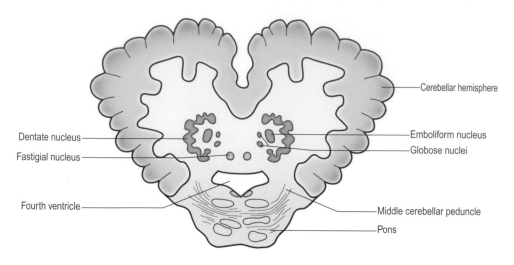

Figure 11.8 **Horizontal section through the cerebellum and brain stem at the level of the fourth ventricle, showing the cerebellar nuclei.**

Figure 11.9 **(A–C) Transverse sections of cerebellar folia showing the layers of the cerebellar cortex.**

- fastigial nucleus
- globose nucleus
- emboliform nucleus
- dentate nucleus (Figs 11.6, 11.7, 11.8).

The dentate nucleus is by far the largest of the cerebellar nuclei and is the only one that can be discerned clearly with the naked eye (Fig. 11.6). It consists of a thin layer of nerve cells folded into a crinkled bag; as a result, it appears somewhat similar to the inferior olivary nucleus of the medulla, from which it receives afferent fibres. The cerebellar nuclei also receive extracerebellar afferents from the vestibular nuclei, reticular nuclei, pontine nuclei and spinocerebellar tracts, predominantly by means of collaterals of mossy fibres destined for the cerebellar cortex. From within the cerebellum, the nuclei receive dense innervation from the Purkinje cells of the cerebellar cortex itself. The cerebellar nuclei constitute the primary source of efferent fibres from the cerebellum to other parts of the brain. The principal destinations of efferent fibres are the reticular and vestibular nuclei of the medulla and pons, the red nucleus of the midbrain and the ventral lateral nucleus of the thalamus.

Internal structure of the cerebellum

- Internally, the cerebellum consists of a surface layer of cortex, highly convoluted to form folia, beneath which lies white matter.
- Within the white matter lie cerebellar nuclei (fastigial, globose, emboliform and dentate).
- The nuclei are the origin of cerebellar efferent fibres.

Functional anatomy of the cerebellum

The cerebellum is often regarded as consisting of three functional subdivisions, based upon phylogenetic, anatomical and functional considerations (Fig. 11.5).

- The **archicerebellum**, or oldest portion in phylogenetic terms, is equated with the **flocculonodular lobe** and the associated **fastigial** nuclei.
- The **paleocerebellum** approximates to the midline **vermis** and surrounding **paravermis**, together with the **globose** and **emboliform** nuclei.
- The **neocerebellum** comprises the remainder (and vast majority) of the **cerebellar hemisphere** and the **dentate nuclei**.

Archicerebellum

The archicerebellum is primarily concerned with the maintenance of balance (equilibrium). It has extensive connections with the vestibular and reticular nuclei of the brain stem, through the inferior cerebellar peduncles (Fig. 11.11). Vestibular information is carried from the vestibular nuclei to the cortex of the ipsilateral flocculonodular lobe. Cortical efferent (Purkinje cell) fibres project to the fastigial nucleus which, in turn, projects back to the vestibular nuclei and to the reticular formation. A significant proportion of fastigial efferents cross to the contralateral side of the brain stem. The influence of the archicerebellum upon the lower motor system is, therefore, bilateral and principally mediated by means of descending vestibulospinal and reticulospinal projections.

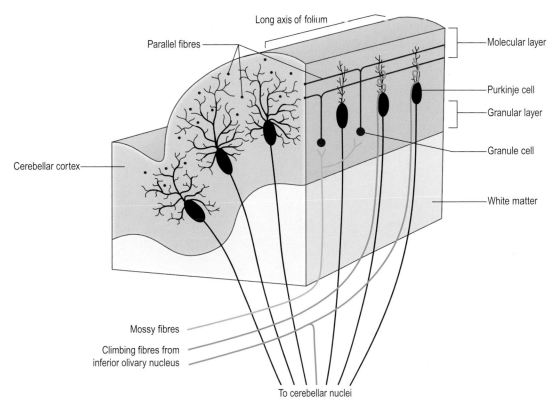

Figure 11.10 **The cerebellar cortex.** Diagram shows afferent and efferent connections and their relationships to the principal cells of the cerebellar cortex.

Paleocerebellum

The paleocerebellum influences muscle tone and posture. Afferents consist principally of dorsal and ventral spinocerebellar tract neurones that carry information from muscle, joint and cutaneous receptors and enter the cerebellum through the inferior and superior cerebellar peduncles, respectively (Fig. 11.12). Fibres terminate largely in the cortex of the ipsilateral vermis and adjacent paravermis. Cerebellar cortical efferents from these areas pass to the globose and emboliform nuclei and also to the fastigial nucleus. The globose and emboliform nuclei project via the superior cerebellar peduncle to the contralateral red nucleus of the midbrain, where they influence the activity of cells giving rise to the descending rubrospinal tract.

Neocerebellum

The neocerebellum is concerned with muscular coordination, including the trajectory, speed and force of movements. The principal afferent pathway consists of pontocerebellar fibres (Fig. 11.13). These originate in the pontine nuclei of the basal portion of the pons and cross to the opposite side, entering the cerebellum through its middle peduncle. Pontocerebellar neurones are influenced by widespread regions of the cerebral cortex involved in the planning and execution of movement. Pontocerebellar fibres terminate predominantly in the lateral parts of the cerebellar hemisphere. Output from the neocerebellar cortex is directed to the dentate nucleus. The dentate nucleus, in turn, projects to the contralateral red nucleus

Reticular nuclei
Fastigial nucleus
Vestibular nuclei
Purkinje cell
Vestibulocerebellar fibres
Vestibular nerve
Reticulospinal and vestibulospinal tracts

Figure 11.11 **Connections of the archicerebellum.** Contralateral projections of the fastigial nucleus are not shown.

Ventral tegmental decussation
Globose and emboliform nuclei
Red nucleus
Decussation of superior cerebellar peduncle
Purkinje cell
Dorsal spinocerebellar tract
Ventral spinocerebellar tract
Rubrospinal tract

Figure 11.12 **Connections of the paleocerebellum.**

and ventral lateral nucleus of the thalamus. The dentate is the largest of the cerebellar nuclei and its efferents form the major part of the superior cerebellar peduncle. The ascending fibres decussate in the caudal midbrain just before reaching the red nucleus. Some relay in the red nucleus with rubrothalamic cells but most bypass the red nucleus and pass directly to the ventral lateral thalamus.

The ventral lateral nucleus of the thalamus projects to the cerebral cortex, particularly the motor cortex of the frontal lobe. The neocerebellum thus exerts its coordinating role in movement primarily through an action on cerebral cortical areas, giving rise to descending corticospinal and corticobulbar pathways.

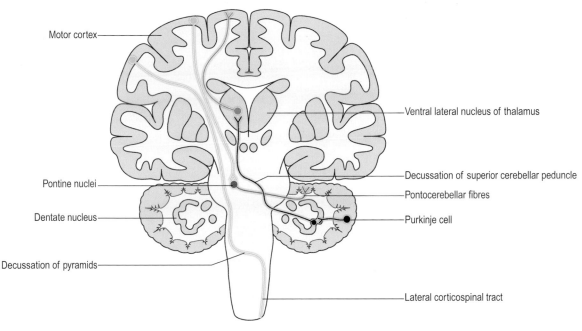

Figure 11.13 **Connections of the neocerebellum.**

Functional anatomy of the cerebellum

- The archicerebellum corresponds to the flocculonodular lobe and fastigial nucleus. Its principal connections are with the vestibular and reticular nuclei of the brain stem and it is concerned with the maintenance of equilibrium.
- The paleocerebellum corresponds to the vermis and paravermal area, together with the globose and emboliform nuclei. It receives fibres from the spinocerebellar tracts and projects to the red nucleus of the midbrain.

- The neocerebellum corresponds to most of the cerebellar hemisphere and the dentate nucleus. It receives afferents from the pons and projects to the ventral lateral nucleus of the thalamus.
- Cerebellar lesions cause incoordination of the upper limbs (intention tremor), lower limbs (cerebellar ataxia), speech (dysarthria) and eyes (nystagmus).

Lesions of the cerebellum

A midline lesion of the cerebellum (such as a tumour) leads to loss of postural control; as a result it is impossible to stand or sit without toppling over, despite preserved coordination of the limbs.

Because of the pattern of ipsilateral and decussated pathways that enter and leave the cerebellum, unilateral lesions of the cerebellar hemisphere cause symptoms on the same side of the body. This is in contrast to cerebral lesions (e.g. in the cerebral cortex, internal capsule or basal ganglia), which give rise to contralateral symptoms.

A unilateral cerebellar hemispheric lesion causes ipsilateral incoordination of the arm (**intention tremor**) and of the leg, causing an unsteady gait, in the absence of weakness or sensory loss.

Bilateral dysfunction of the cerebellum, caused by alcoholic intoxication, hypothyroidism, inherited cerebellar degeneration/ataxia, multiple sclerosis or paraneoplastic disease, causes slowness and slurring of speech (**dysarthria**), incoordination of both arms and a staggering, wide-based, unsteady gait (**cerebellar ataxia**).

Cerebellar lesions also impair coordination of eye movements and the eyes exhibit a to-and-fro motion (**nystagmus**), greatest in amplitude when gaze is directed to the same side as the lesion. Nystagmus is a very common feature of multiple sclerosis. The combination of nystagmus with dysarthria and intention tremor constitutes 'Charcot's triad', which is highly diagnostic of the disease.

Chapter 12
Thalamus

Rostral to the midbrain lies the forebrain (prosencephalon, cerebrum; Fig. 1.10). The forebrain consists of the bilaterally paired diencephalon and cerebral hemisphere on each side and is by far the largest derivative of the three basic embryological divisions of the brain (pp. 5–6). The diencephalon is continuous with the rostral part of the midbrain and lies between the brain stem and the cerebral hemisphere. The diencephalon is comprised of – from dorsal to ventral: the epithalamus, thalamus, subthalamus and hypothalamus, of which the thalamus is the largest. The **thalamus** consists of numerous nuclei, most of which have extensive reciprocal connections with the cerebral cortex. Of particular note are:

- nuclei that transmit general and special sensory information to corresponding regions of the sensory cortices
- nuclei that receive impulses from the cerebellum and basal ganglia and interface with motor regions of the frontal lobe
- nuclei that have connections with associative and limbic areas of the cerebral cortex.

The diencephalon is almost entirely surrounded by the cerebral hemisphere; consequently, little of its structure can be seen externally, apart from the ventral portion of the **hypothalamus**, which can be seen on the base of the brain (Fig. 12.1). Immediately caudal to the optic chiasma is a small midline elevation, the **tuber cinereum**. From its apex extends the **infundibulum** or pituitary stalk, which attaches to the pituitary gland. Caudal to the tuber cinereum, a pair of rounded eminences, the mammillary bodies, are located on either side of the midline. These contain the mammillary nuclei of the hypothalamus. The hypothalamus lies below the thalamus, extending medial and ventral to the subthalamus. It has important connections with the limbic system, a controlling influence upon the activity of the autonomic nervous system and a central role in neuroendocrine function, partly through its relationship with the pituitary gland. The hypothalamus is discussed further in Chapter 16.

The other parts of the diencephalon can be seen in sagittal and coronal sections of the brain (Figs 12.2, 12.3). The diencephalon forms the lateral wall of the third ventricle. The dorsal part of the ventricular wall is formed by the thalamus and the ventral part by the hypothalamus. The **epithalamus** is a relatively small part of the diencephalon located in its most caudal and dorsal region, immediately rostral to the superior colliculus of the midbrain. It consists principally of the **pineal gland** and the **habenula** (**habenular nuclei**). The pineal gland is an endocrine organ. It synthesises the hormone melatonin. The pineal gland has been implicated in control of the sleep/waking cycle (circadian rhythm) and in regulation of the onset of puberty. The habenular nuclei have connections with the limbic system (Ch. 16).

The **subthalamus** lies beneath the thalamus and dorsolateral to the hypothalamus, with its ventrolateral aspect against the internal capsule. It contains two notable cell groups, the **subthalamic nucleus** and the **zona incerta**. The subthalamic nucleus is located in the ventrolateral part of the subthalamus, immediately medial to the internal capsule. It has the shape of a biconvex lens in coronal section. The subthalamic nucleus has prominent connections with the globus pallidus and the substantia nigra and is important in the control of movement. It is discussed in more detail in Chapter 14. The zona incerta is a rostral extension of the brain stem reticular formation. Several important fibre systems traverse the subthalamus *en route* to the thalamus. These include ascending sensory projections (medial lemniscus, spinothalamic tracts, trigeminothalamic tracts), cerebellothalamic fibres from the dentate nucleus and pallidothalamic fibres from the medial segment of the globus pallidus. The last envelop the zona incerta as the lenticular fasciculus and thalamic fasciculus (see Fig. 14.8).

Topographical anatomy of the thalamus

External features
The thalamus has been likened in size and shape to a small hen's egg. Together with the hypothalamus it forms the lateral wall of the third ventricle, the transition between the two being marked by a faint groove, the hypothalamic sulcus. In most individuals, the two thalami are joined across the thin slit of the ventricle by the **interthalamic adhesion** or **massa intermedia**. A fascicle of nerve fibres, the **stria medullaris**, which has limbic connections, courses along the dorsomedial margin of the thalamus (Fig. 12.2). Along this line, the ependymal lining of the third ventricle spans the narrow lumen to form the ventricular roof.

Optic nerve

Infundibulum

Tuber cinereum

Oculomotor nerve

Optic chiasma

Optic tract

Crus cerebri

Mammillary body

Figure 12.1 **Ventral aspect of the diencephalon.**

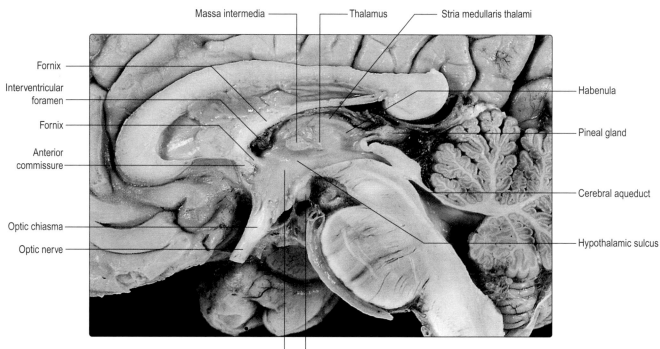

Massa intermedia — Thalamus — Stria medullaris thalami

Fornix

Interventricular
foramen

Fornix

Anterior
commissure

Optic chiasma

Optic nerve

Habenula

Pineal gland

Cerebral aqueduct

Hypothalamic sulcus

Hypothalamus — Mammillary body

Figure 12.2 **Median sagittal section of the brain showing the relationships of the diencephalon.**

The anterior pole of the thalamus extends as far as the interventricular foramen, through which the third and lateral ventricles are in continuity. Lateral to the thalamus lies the posterior limb of the internal capsule and anterolateral lies the head of the caudate nucleus (Fig. 12.4). The dorsal aspect of the thalamus thus forms part of the floor of the body of the lateral ventricle. Another fascicle of nerve fibres with limbic connections, the **stria terminalis**, marks the boundary between thalamus and caudate (Fig. 12.4). Ventral to the thalamus lie the subthalamus and hypothalamus; caudal to it lies the midbrain.

Internal organisation
Within the thalamus is located a thin layer of nerve fibres composed of some of the afferent and efferent connections of thalamic nuclei. This is called the **internal medullary lamina** (Figs 12.3, 12.5, 12.6). The lamina is roughly Y-shaped when viewed from above and provides the basis for dividing the main part of the thalamus into three nuclear masses: **anterior**, **medial** and **lateral**. Each of these cellular complexes is further subdivided into a number of individually named nuclei. Embedded within the internal medullary lamina are several cell groups, known collectively as the **intralaminar nuclei** (Figs 12.5, 12.6). Lateral to the main mass of thalamic nuclei lies another sheet of nerve fibres, the **lateral medullary lamina**, which consists of thalamocortical and corticothalamic fibres. Between this and the internal capsule is located a thin stratum of neurones that constitute the **reticular nucleus** of the thalamus (Fig. 12.3).

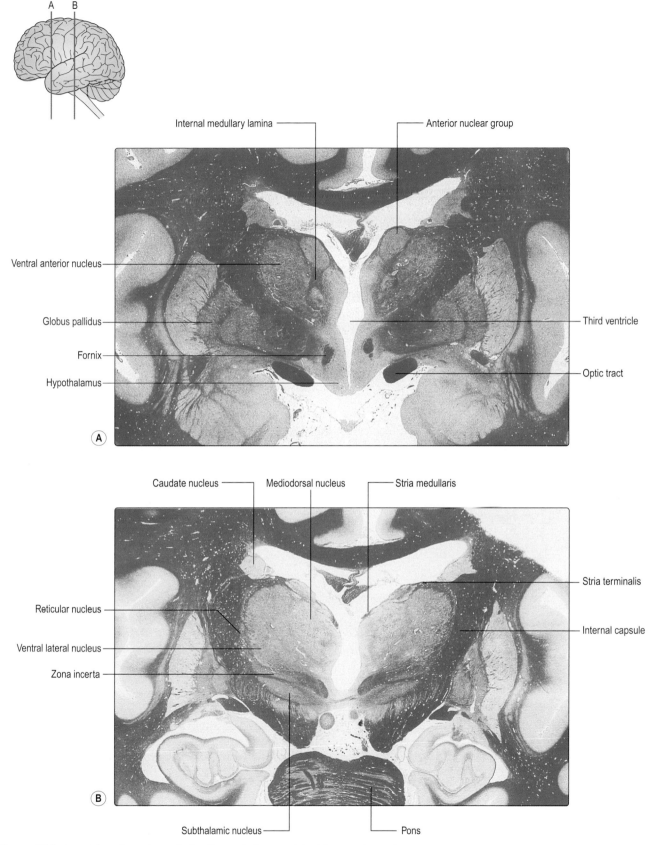

Figure 12.3 **Coronal sections through the diencephalon.** Luxol fast blue stain for myelin.

Anatomy of the thalamus

- The thalamus is the largest component of the diencephalon, which is situated between the brain stem and the cerebral hemisphere.
- Almost all thalamic nuclei have rich reciprocal connections with the cerebral cortex.
- The thalamus is divided into three principal nuclear masses (anterior, medial and lateral) by the internal medullary lamina.

- Embedded within the internal medullary lamina lie intralaminar nuclei.
- On the lateral aspect of the thalamus lies the thin reticular nucleus.

Corpus callosum — Frontal lobe — Head of caudate nucleus

Choroid plexus
of lateral ventricle
overlying thalamus — Fornix — Occipital lobe — Stria terminalis

Figure 12.4 **Dorsal aspect of the diencephalon.** The choroid plexus has been removed on the right side.

Functional organisation of thalamic nuclei

All the nuclei of the thalamus, with the exception of the reticular nucleus, project to the ipsilateral cerebral cortex and the whole of the cortex receives input from the thalamus. Similarly, all thalamic nuclei receive corticofugal fibres in a basically reciprocal fashion. In some cases, precise, point-to-point projections exist between individual thalamic nuclei and restricted cortical zones with well-defined sensory or motor functions. This typifies the relationship between the thalamic nuclei and cortical regions that subserve the general and special senses and the motor regions that receive cerebellar and basal ganglia input (Fig. 12.6).

Such thalamic nuclei are often referred to as the 'specific' nuclei. The specific nuclei all lie within the ventral part (tier) of the lateral nuclear group. Other thalamic nuclei receive less functionally distinct afferent input that does not include overtly sensory or motor pathways; in turn, these

connect with wider areas of cortex, including associative and limbic domains. These are often referred to as the 'non-specific' nuclei. Non-specific thalamic nuclei include the nuclei of the dorsal tier of the lateral nuclear complex as well as the whole of the anterior and medial complexes.

> ### Thalamic lesions
> Strokes and tumours destroying the thalamus lead to loss of sensation in the contralateral face and limbs, accompanied by a distressing discomfort in the paradoxically anaesthetic areas (**thalamic pain**).
>
> Thalamic lesions may mimic focal cortical defects because of the richness of thalamocortical connections.

Lateral nuclear group

The lateral nuclear group contains all of the so-called 'specific' thalamic nuclei. These are located in the ventral part of the complex and include the ventral anterior, ventral lateral, ventral posterior, lateral geniculate and medial geniculate nuclei (Figs 12.5, 12.6).

Ventral posterior nucleus

The ventral posterior (VP) nucleus lies between the ventrolateral nucleus and the pulvinar. Within the ventral posterior nucleus there is termination of all the ascending pathways from the spinal cord and brain stem that carry general sensory information from the contralateral half of the body to a conscious level. These pathways include the spinothalamic tracts, medial lemniscus and trigeminothalamic tracts. The termination of these fibres in the ventral posterior nucleus is highly organised somatotopically.

An extensive, lateral portion of the nucleus receives information from the trunk and limbs via the spinothalamic tracts and medial lemniscus. This is referred to as the ventral posterolateral (VPl) division (Fig. 12.6). A smaller, medial portion of the ventral posterior nucleus receives information from the head, via the trigeminothalamic tract, and is termed the ventral posteromedial nucleus (VPm). This area also receives taste information from the nucleus solitarius of the medulla and vestibular information from the vestibular nuclei. The ventral posterior nucleus projects to the primary somatosensory cortex in the postcentral gyrus of the parietal lobe.

Lateral geniculate nucleus

The geniculate nuclei are located near the posterior pole of the thalamus, ventral to the pulvinar. Here they form small eminences on the surface, known as the geniculate bodies. The lateral geniculate nucleus is a part of the visual system and receives further discussion in Chapter 15. It is the site of termination of the optic tract, which carries the axons of retinal ganglion cells. As a result of hemidecussation of optic nerve fibres in the optic chiasma, each nucleus receives axons that have originated in the ipsilateral temporal hemiretina and the contralateral nasal hemiretina and is thus provided with visual information relating to the

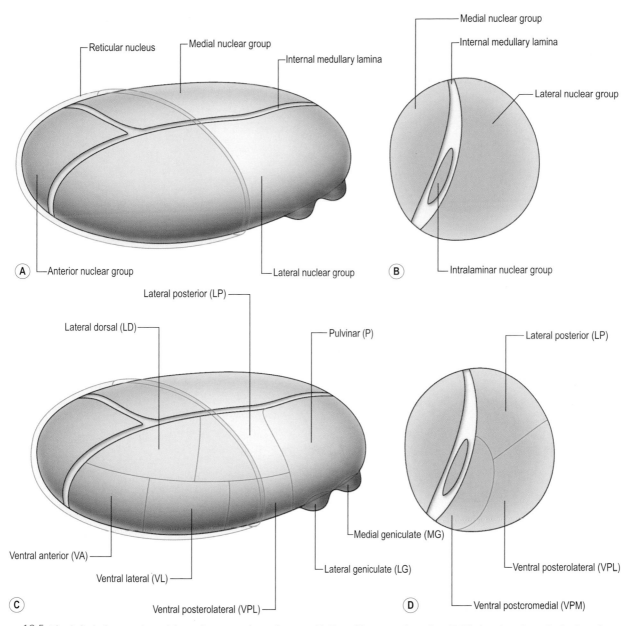

Figure 12.5 **The left thalamus viewed from the anterolateral aspect (A,C) and in coronal section (B,D) showing the principal nuclear groups (A,B) and the divisions of the lateral nuclear group (C,D).**

contralateral half of the visual field. The lateral geniculate nucleus sends fibres, via the retrolenticular part of the internal capsule and the optic radiation, to the primary visual cortex of the occipital lobe.

Medial geniculate nucleus

The medial geniculate nucleus is part of the auditory system, which is described in Chapter 10. It receives ascending fibres from the inferior colliculus of the midbrain, via the inferior brachium. The medial geniculate nucleus projects, via the retrolenticular part of the internal capsule and the auditory radiation, to the primary auditory cortex of the temporal lobe.

Ventral anterior nucleus

The ventral anterior (VA) nucleus occupies the rostral part of the lateral nuclear mass. It consists of two subdivisions: the larger, principal part (VApc) and the smaller, magnocellular part (VAmc). The principal subcortical afferents to this region are output fibres of the ipsilateral

basal ganglia system, which originate from the medial segment of the globus pallidus and its homologue, the pars reticulata of the substantia nigra. Fibres from the globus pallidus terminate in VApc, while those from the substantia nigra end in VAmc. The ventral anterior nucleus of the thalamus has reciprocal connections with motor regions of the frontal lobe, particularly the premotor and supplementary motor cortices. It is, therefore, an important part of the mechanism by which the basal ganglia exert their influence on normal movement and through which abnormalities of movement are mediated in basal ganglia disorders.

Ventral lateral nucleus

The ventral lateral (VL) nucleus lies immediately caudal to the ventral anterior nucleus in the ventral tier of the lateral nuclear complex. It consists of three subdivisions: pars oralis (VLo), pars medialis (VLm) and pars caudalis (VLc). Subcortical afferents to the ventral lateral nucleus originate mainly from the ipsilateral globus pallidus and substantia

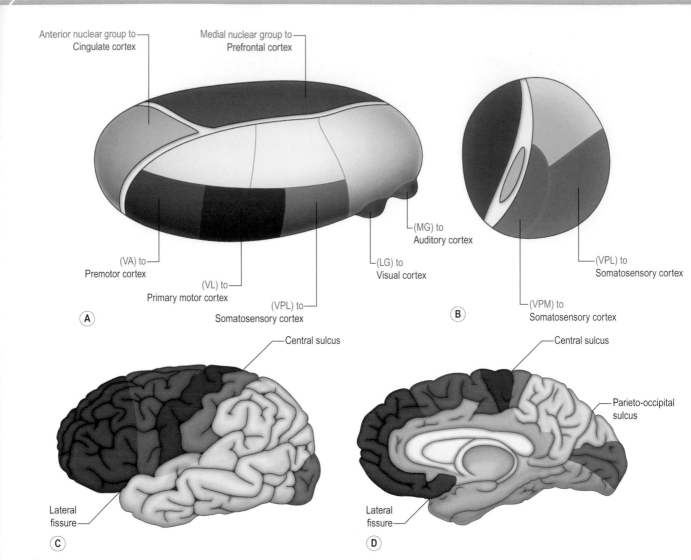

Figure 12.6 **Organisation of thalamic nuclei and their principal relationships with the cerebral cortex.** The thalamus is viewed from its anterolateral aspect **(A)** and in coronal section **(B)**. Colours indicate the relationships between thalamic nuclei and corresponding cerebral cortical regions on the lateral **(C)** and medial **(D)** aspects of the cerebral hemisphere.

nigra, and from the contralateral dentate nucleus of the cerebellum. Pallidal and nigral afferents terminate in VLo and VLm, while those from the cerebellum terminate in VLc. The ventral lateral nucleus, like the ventral anterior nucleus, has reciprocal connections with motor areas of the frontal lobe and especially with the primary motor cortex of the precentral gyrus.

Surgical treatment of disorders of the basal ganglia and cerebellum

Neurosurgically placed lesions in the region of the ventral anterior and ventral lateral nuclei have been used to alleviate some of the motor symptoms associated with disorders of the basal ganglia (rigidity, tremor at rest, dyskinesias) and cerebellum (intention tremor). Such **thalamotomy** has been largely superseded by drug therapy in basal ganglia disease but is still used to relieve cerebellar tremor, e.g. in multiple sclerosis.

Functional organisation of the lateral nuclear group

- 'Specific' thalamic nuclei have well-defined sensory or motor functions and highly organised connections with sensory and motor regions of the cerebral cortex. They all lie within the ventral tier of the lateral nuclear mass and include:
  - Ventral posterior nucleus: receives general sensory afferents in the medial lemniscus, spinothalamic tract and trigeminothalamic tract; sends efferents to the primary somatosensory cortex of the parietal lobe.
  - Lateral geniculate nucleus: receives visual afferents in the optic tract; projects to the primary visual cortex of the occipital lobe.
  - Medial geniculate nucleus: receives auditory afferents from the inferior colliculus; sends efferents to the primary auditory cortex of the temporal lobe.
  - Ventral anterior and ventral lateral nuclei: receive afferents from the cerebellum and basal ganglia; send efferents to motor cortical areas of the frontal lobe.
- 'Non-specific' nuclei connect with wider areas of cortex, including associative and limbic regions.

Within the dorsal tier of the lateral nuclear complex lie a number of so-called 'non-specific' nuclei. Among these, the lateral dorsal nucleus is part of the limbic system. It receives afferents from the hippocampus and sends efferents to the cingulate gyrus. The lateral posterior nucleus has connections with the sensory association cortex of the parietal lobe. The **pulvinar** is a large region at the most posterior part of the thalamus. It has extensive connections with association cortices of the parietal, temporal and occipital lobes.

Anterior nuclear group

The most anterior portion of the thalamus, extending to its rostral pole, is the anterior nuclear complex. It consists of three subdivisions: the anteroventral, anteromedial and anterodorsal nuclei. The individual connections of these will not be discussed. The anterior nuclear group is part of the limbic system. It receives a large afferent projection from the mammillary body of the hypothalamus via the mammillothalamic tract. The anterior complex projects principally to the cingulate gyrus on the medial surface of the cerebral hemisphere (Fig. 16.11). It is involved in the control of instinctive drives, in the emotional aspects of behaviour and in memory.

Medial nuclear group

The medial nuclear group forms a large region consisting primarily of the mediodorsal nucleus (dorsomedial nucleus) and some much smaller components, such as the nucleus reuniens. Subcortical afferents to the mediodorsal nucleus come from the hypothalamus, amygdala and from other thalamic nuclei, including the intralaminar nuclei and nuclei of the lateral complex. Extensive reciprocal connections exist between the mediodorsal nucleus and the prefrontal cortex. It is concerned mainly with the control of mood and the emotions.

Intralaminar nuclei

Several nuclei lie embedded within the internal medullary lamina of the thalamus. These include the centromedian and parafascicular nuclei, the centromedian being the largest intralaminar nucleus in humans. The intralaminar nuclei receive ascending afferents from the brain stem reticular formation and also from the spinothalamic and trigeminothalamic systems. In turn, they project to widespread regions of the cerebral cortex and to the caudate nucleus and putamen of the basal ganglia. The intralaminar nuclei are part of the mechanism for activation of the cerebral cortical mantle. When they are stimulated, alpha rhythm activity, which is associated with repose and sleep, is disrupted and the electroencephalogram (EEG) becomes desynchronised. Lesions of the intralaminar nuclei reduce the perception of pain and the level of consciousness.

Reticular nucleus

The reticular nucleus is a thin layer of cells located on the lateral aspect of the thalamus between the external medullary lamina and the internal capsule. This nucleus receives collaterals of both thalamocortical and corticothalamic fibres, which pass between other thalamic nuclei and the cerebral cortex.

Functional organisation of anterior, medial, intralaminar and reticular nuclei

- The anterior nuclear group of the thalamus is part of the limbic system. This region receives fibres from the mammillary body of the hypothalamus and projects to the cingulate gyrus.
- Within the medial nuclear group, the mediodorsal nucleus has extensive reciprocal connections with the cortex of the frontal lobe.
- The intralaminar nuclei receive input from the reticular formation and ascending sensory systems. They project to the cerebral cortex and the striatum and are responsible for activation of the cerebral cortex.
- The reticular nucleus receives collaterals of thalamocortical and corticothalamic fibres.

Chapter 13
Cerebral hemisphere and cerebral cortex

The cerebral hemisphere is derived from the embryological telencephalon (Ch. 1). It is the largest part of the forebrain and it reaches the greatest degree of development in the human brain. Superficially, the cerebral hemisphere consists of a layer of grey matter, the cerebral cortex, which is highly convoluted to form a complex pattern of ridges (gyri) and furrows (sulci). This serves to maximise the surface area of the cerebral cortex, about 70% of which is hidden within the depths of sulci (Figs 13.1, 13.2). Beneath the surface, axons running to and from the cells of the cortex form an extensive mass of white matter. Figures 13.3–13.12 show successive coronal sections through the brain. The vast majority of those nerve fibres that pass between the cerebral cortex and subcortical structures are condensed, deep within the hemisphere, into a broad sheet called the **internal capsule** (Figs 13.4–13.11; see also Fig. 1.23). Between the internal capsule and the cortical surface, fibres radiate in and out to produce a fan-like arrangement, the **corona radiata**. Buried within the white matter lie a number of nuclear masses. Most notable among these are the caudate nucleus, putamen and globus pallidus, known collectively as the corpus striatum or basal ganglia (Figs 13.3–13.15). Within the cerebral hemisphere lies the large C-shaped cavity of the lateral ventricle, which is considered with the rest of the ventricular system in Chapter 6.

The two cerebral hemispheres are separated by a deep cleft, the **great longitudinal fissure**, which accommodates the meningeal **falx cerebri**. In the depths of the fissure, the hemispheres are united by the **corpus callosum**, an enormous sheet of commissural nerve fibres which run between corresponding areas of the two cortices (Figs 13.2–13.15; see also Figs 13.22, 13.23, 13.24).

Gyri, sulci and lobes of the cerebral hemisphere

Certain gyri and sulci on the surface of the hemisphere are consistently located in different individuals and form the basis of dividing the hemisphere into four lobes, namely the **frontal**, **parietal**, **temporal** and **occipital lobes**. Their

principal topographical features and functional significance are described below. The most conspicuous and deepest cleft on the lateral surface of the hemisphere is the **lateral fissure** (Fig. 13.1). This separates the temporal lobe below, from the frontal and parietal lobes above. Within the depths of the lateral fissure lies a cortical area known as the **insula** (Figs 13.6–13.14). The parts of the frontal, parietal and temporal lobes that overlie the insula are called the **opercula**. Also on the lateral surface of the hemisphere, a single, uninterrupted sulcus can usually be identified, running continuously between the great longitudinal fissure and the lateral fissure. This is the **central sulcus**, which marks the boundary between the frontal and parietal lobes (Figs 13.1, 13.16). The central sulcus extends for a short distance onto the medial surface of the hemisphere, within the great longitudinal fissure (Figs 13.2, 13.16).

The frontal lobe constitutes the entire region in front of the central sulcus. Immediately in front of the sulcus, and running parallel to it, lies the **precentral gyrus**, which is the primary motor region of the cerebral cortex. In front of the precentral gyrus, the rest of the frontal lobe consists of a more variable pattern of convolutions, of which the **superior**, **middle** and **inferior frontal gyri** can usually be identified (Fig. 13.1).

Behind the central sulcus, and above the lateral fissure, lies the parietal lobe. Its most anterior part is the **postcentral gyrus**, which is the site of the primary somatosensory cortex. Behind the postcentral gyrus, on the lateral surface of the hemisphere, the **intraparietal sulcus** divides the rest of the parietal lobe into superior and inferior parietal lobules (Figs 13.1, 13.16).

The boundary between the parietal lobe and the posteriorly located occipital lobe is not coincident with a single sulcus on the lateral surface of the hemisphere; however, it is clearly marked by the deep **parieto-occipital sulcus** on the medial surface (Figs 13.2, 13.16). The occipital lobe does not bear any important landmarks on its lateral surface but, on the medial surface, the prominent **calcarine sulcus** indicates the location of the primary visual cortex (Figs 13.2, 13.16).

The temporal lobe lies beneath the lateral fissure, merging posteriorly with the parietal and occipital lobes. On its lateral surface the temporal lobe is divided into three principal gyri that run roughly parallel to the lateral fissure: the **superior**, **middle** and **inferior temporal gyri** (Fig. 13.1). The superior temporal gyrus includes the primary auditory cortex. Most of this functional region is situated on the superior bank of the gyrus, within the lateral fissure, where the **transverse temporal gyri**, or **Heschl's convolutions**, provide a more precise localisation (Fig. 13.17).

Figure 13.1 **Lateral aspect of the cerebral hemisphere showing major gyri and sulci.**

Figure 13.2 **Median sagittal section of the cerebral hemisphere showing major gyri and sulci.** The brain stem and cerebellum have been removed to show the inferomedial aspect of the temporal lobe.

Figure 13.3 **Coronal section of the cerebral hemisphere.**

Head of caudate nucleus

Anterior limb of internal capsule

Figure 13.4 **Coronal section of the cerebral hemisphere.**

Anterior horn of lateral ventricle

Temporal lobe

Corpus callosum

Septum pellucidum

Figure 13.5 **Coronal section of the cerebral hemisphere.**

Anterior limb of internal capsule

Nucleus accumbens

Septum pellucidum

Caudate nucleus

Putamen

Septum

Figure 13.6 **Coronal section of the cerebral hemisphere.**

Corona radiata

Extreme capsule

External capsule

Putamen

Globus pallidus

Internal capsule

Insula

Anterior commissure

Anterior column of fornix

Substantia innominata

Figure 13.7 **Coronal section of the cerebral hemisphere.**

Caudate nucleus

Lateral medullary lamina

Globus pallidus { external segment / internal segment }

Amygdala

Mammillary body

Lateral fissure

Fornix

Claustrum

Hippocampus

Figure 13.8 **Coronal section of the cerebral hemisphere.**

Insula

Tail of caudate nucleus

Hippocampus

Subthalamic nucleus

Internal capsule

Thalamus

Third ventricle

Substantia nigra

Figure 13.9 **Coronal section of the cerebral hemisphere.**

Great longitudinal fissure

Fornix

Inferior horn of
lateral ventricle

Crus cerebri

Substantia nigra

Thalamus

Red nucleus

Figure 13.10 **Coronal section of the cerebral hemisphere.**

Lateral fissure

Tail of caudate nucleus

Temporal lobe

Lateral geniculate nucleus

Habenula

Posterior
commissure

Pons

Figure 13.11 **Coronal section of the cerebral hemisphere.**

Pulvinar

Hippocampus

Brachium conjunctivum

Fornix

Pineal gland

Pedunculopontine nucleus

Cerebral aqueduct

Figure 13.12 **Coronal section of the cerebral hemisphere.**

Figure 13.13 **Horizontal (axial) magnetic resonance image of the living brain.** (Courtesy of Professor A Jackson, Wolfson Molecular Imaging Centre, University of Manchester, Manchester, UK.)

Figure 13.14 **Horizontal section of the brain.**

Figure 13.15 **Coronal magnetic resonance image of the living brain.** (Courtesy of Professor A Jackson, Wolfson Molecular Imaging Centre, University of Manchester, Manchester, UK.)

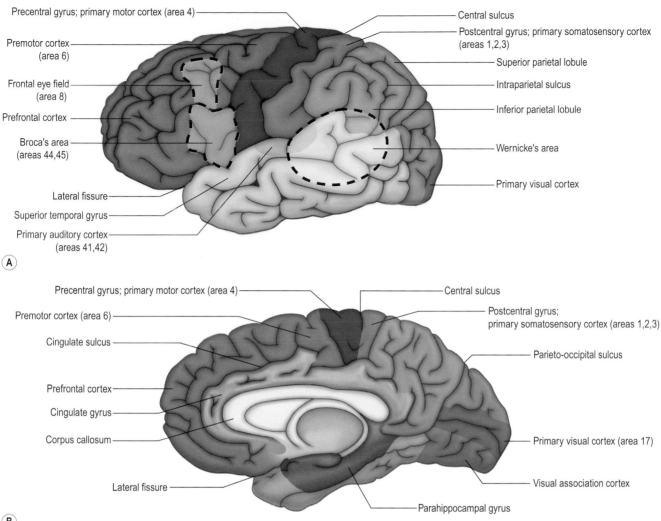

Figure 13.16 **Major functional areas of the cerebral cortex: (A)** Lateral aspect of left cerebral hemisphere; **(B)** Medial aspect of right cerebral hemisphere in sagittal section.

Figure 13.17 **Superolateral aspect of the left cerebral hemisphere.** The frontal and parietal operculae have been removed to show the location of the transverse temporal gyri (Heschl's convolutions) and the insula.

On the medial surface of the hemisphere, certain portions of the frontal, parietal and temporal lobes also constitute components of the limbic system. Curving around the corpus callosum, and running parallel to it, lies the **cingulate gyrus** (Figs 13.2, 13.16), separated from the rest of the hemisphere by the **cingulate sulcus**. The cingulate gyrus passes posteriorly and inferiorly round the posterior portion, or splenium, of the corpus callosum to become continuous with the **parahippocampal gyrus** of the temporal lobe. Deep to the parahippocampal gyrus, within the temporal lobe, lies the **hippocampus** (Figs 13.8–13.12). This structure is formed by an in-curling of the inferomedial part of the temporal lobe. The cingulate gyrus, parahippocampal gyrus and hippocampus are sometimes referred to as the **limbic lobe** of the cerebral hemisphere.

Gyri, sulci and lobes of the cerebral hemisphere

- The cerebral hemisphere consists of:
  - The superficial cerebral cortex, convoluted to form gyri and sulci
  - Underlying white matter, consisting of cortical afferent and efferent fibres
  - Deep nuclear masses, the basal ganglia.
- The two cerebral hemispheres are separated by the great longitudinal fissure and joined by the corpus callosum.
- The hemisphere is divided into four lobes (frontal, parietal, temporal and occipital) on the basis of surface topography.
- Principal landmarks that indicate the divisions between lobes are the lateral fissure, central sulcus and parieto-occipital sulcus.

Figure 13.18 **The histological structure of the cerebral cortex.** (From Mitchell, G A G and Patterson, E L. Basic Anatomy. London: Livingstone; 1954. Courtesy of Churchill Livingstone.)

Cerebral cortex

Histological structure

The cerebral cortex forms the outer surface of the cerebral hemisphere. It consists of a layer, several millimetres in thickness, of nerve cell bodies, dendritic arborisations and synaptic interconnections. In the early part of the twentieth century, the Swedish anatomist Brodmann produced a numbered, cytoarchitectural map of the cerebral cortex based upon its regional histological characteristics. Although largely superseded by the elucidation of function, in some instances there is good correspondence between **Brodmann's areas** and functionally defined regions of the cortex. In such cases, Brodmann's numbers are retained in common use for descriptive purposes.

Long ago in evolutionary history, the cerebral cortex originally arose in relation to olfactory function. Phylogenetically old parts of the cortex (referred to as **archicortex** and **paleocortex**), such as the hippocampus and other parts of the temporal lobe, retain throughout evolution an association with the olfactory system and have a primitive, three-layered cytoarchitecture. These regions have important functions in the emotional aspects of behaviour and in memory. Together with other parts of the cortex and certain subcortical nuclei they constitute the limbic system (Ch. 16). However, most of the cerebral cortex is a more recent acquisition in phylogenetic terms and is referred to as the **neocortex**. Although its detailed

cytological structure varies from region to region, it is generally recognised as consisting of six layers (Fig. 13.18):

- **Layer I**, the most superficial layer, contains few nerve cell bodies but many dendritic and axonal processes in synaptic interaction.
- **Layer II** contains many small neurones, which establish intracortical connections.
- **Layer III** contains medium-sized neurones giving rise to association and commissural fibres.
- **Layer IV** is the site of termination of afferent fibres from the specific thalamic nuclei.
- **Layer V** is the origin of projection fibres to extracortical targets, such as basal ganglia, thalamus, brain stem and spinal cord. In the primary motor cortex of the frontal lobe, this layer contains the giant Betz cells, which project fibres into the pyramidal tract.
- **Layer VI** also contains association and projection neurones.

Functional organisation

The cerebral cortex is necessary for conscious awareness and thought, memory and intellect. It is the region to which all sensory modalities ultimately ascend (mostly via the thalamus) and where they are consciously perceived and interpreted in the light of previous experience. The cerebral cortex is the highest level at which the motor system is represented. It is here that actions are conceived and initiated.

- The posterior part of the cerebrum receives sensory information from the outside world in the primary sensory areas of the parietal lobe (somatosensory), occipital lobe (vision) and temporal lobe (hearing).
- In adjacent cortical zones, the information is elaborated to permit identification of objects by touch, sight and hearing in a modality-specific act of perception. Areas of cortex at the junction of the three cerebral lobes, known as association cortex, are critical for the multimodal and spatial recognition of the environment.
- The medial portions of the cerebral hemisphere (limbic system) enable the storage and retrieval of information processed in the posterior hemispheric regions.
- The anterior part of the cerebrum (frontal lobe) is concerned with the organisation of movement (primary motor area; premotor and supplementary motor areas) and the strategic guidance of complex motor behaviour over time (prefrontal area).
- In the majority of individuals, areas of association cortex in frontal, parietal and temporal lobes of the left hemisphere are responsible for the comprehension and expression of language. The left hemisphere is, therefore, said to be **dominant** for language.

Focal cerebral lesions

Focal cerebral lesions, e.g. a stroke or tumour, produce three kinds of symptom:

1. **Focal epileptic seizures.** The repetitive discharges of groups of neurones in the cerebral cortex produce paroxysmal attacks lasting for brief periods and reflecting the functional properties of the neurones concerned. The patient experiences sudden attacks of abnormal movements or sensations (**simple focal seizures**) or brief alterations in perception, mood and behaviour (**complex partial seizures**). Focal seizures may trigger **generalised (tonic–clonic) seizures**.
2. **Sensory/motor deficits.** There is a loss of sensation or movement, detectable on clinical neurological examination.
3. **Psychological deficits.** There are breakdowns in psychological processes such as language, perception and memory, demonstrable on psychological evaluation.

If the focal lesion is space-occupying, the syndrome of **raised intracranial pressure** results (see p. 47).

A **unilateral cerebral hemisphere lesion** causes mental impairment (e.g. aphasia), a contralateral spastic hemiparesis, hyperreflexia and an extensor plantar response (upper motor neurone lesion), and contralateral hemisensory loss (Fig. 13.19; see also Fig. 1.41). A vascular insult to the internal capsule, such as an infarction or haemorrhage, leads to the rapid development of this syndrome, known as **stroke**.

Frontal lobe

The frontal lobe lies anterior to the central sulcus. Immediately anterior to the central sulcus, and running parallel to it, is the precentral gyrus. Functionally, this is known as the **primary motor cortex** (Figs 13.1, 13.2,

13.16). It corresponds to Brodmann's area 4. Within the cortex of the precentral gyrus, the contralateral half of the body is represented in a precise somatotopic fashion (Fig. 13.20). The representation of the body is inverted, with the head area located in the most inferior part of the precentral gyrus, just above the lateral fissure. Progressing superiorly, successive areas of cortex represent the digits, hand, arm, shoulder and trunk. The lower limb is represented on the medial surface of the hemisphere, above the corpus callosum. The area of cortex devoted to a particular body part is proportional, not to its size, but to the degree of precision with which movements can be executed. Therefore, the larynx, tongue, face and digits of the hand are represented by relatively large regions.

Stimulation of the primary motor cortex elicits contraction of discrete muscle groups on the opposite side of the body. The function of this region is the control of voluntary, skilled movements, sometimes referred to as fractionated movements; 30% of corticospinal (pyramidal tract) and corticobulbar fibres arise from neurones of the primary motor cortex, about 3% originating from giant pyramidal (Betz) cells. The principal subcortical afferents to the primary motor cortex originate from the ventral lateral nucleus of the thalamus (see Fig. 12.6), which in turn receives input mainly from the dentate nucleus of the cerebellum and from the globus pallidus of the basal ganglia.

The region immediately anterior to the primary motor cortex is known as the **premotor cortex** (Brodmann's area 6) (Fig. 13.16). On the lateral surface of the hemisphere, this includes the posterior portions of the superior, middle and inferior frontal gyri. On the medial surface of the hemisphere, the premotor cortex includes a region referred to as the **supplementary motor cortex**. Here, like the primary motor cortex, there is somatotopic representation of the body although, unlike the primary motor cortex, representation appears to be bilateral in both hemispheres.

Stimulation of premotor cortical areas induces movements that are less focused than those elicited from the primary motor cortex and that involve groups of functionally related muscles. Movements evoked from the supplementary motor cortex tend to be postural in nature, involving axial and proximal musculature. Premotor cortical areas are thought to function in the programming of, and preparation for, movement and in the control of posture. The premotor cortex exerts its actions partly via the primary motor cortex, with which it is connected by short association fibres, and partly via corticospinal and corticobulbar fibres. About 30% of the latter originate in the premotor cortex although, unlike the primary motor cortex, giant Betz cells are absent from premotor areas. The principal subcortical input to premotor cortical regions, including the supplementary motor cortex, is the ventral anterior nucleus of the thalamus. This, in turn, receives fibres from the globus pallidus and substantia nigra.

Immediately in front of the premotor cortex, on the lateral surface of the hemisphere, are located two other important regions. In the middle frontal gyrus lies the **frontal eye field** (Brodmann's area 8). This region controls voluntary conjugate deviation of the eyes, as occur when scanning the visual field. Unilateral damage to this area causes conjugate deviation of the eyes towards the side of the lesion. In the inferior frontal gyrus of the dominant

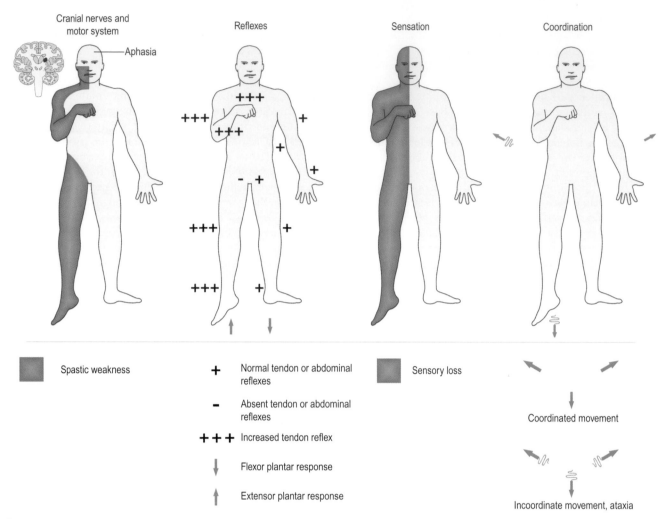

Figure 13.19 **Unilateral cerebral hemisphere lesion.**

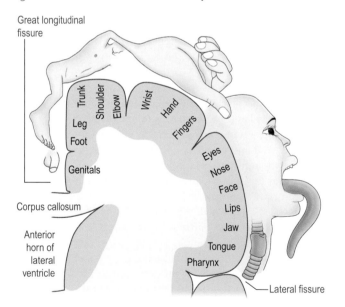

Figure 13.20 **Schematic coronal section through the cerebral hemisphere illustrating the approximate somatotopic representation of the contralateral body half in the motor and sensory cortices.**

Left frontal lobe lesions
Lesions of the left frontal lobe cause:

- Focal seizures. Paroxysmal jerking movements of the contralateral limbs are termed 'simple motor' or **'Jacksonian' seizures**.
- Sensory/motor deficit. Weakness of the face and upper motor neurone signs in the limbs on the opposite side to the lesion occur (**contralateral hemiplegia**).
- Psychological deficit. Speech is produced with great effort and poor articulation, in brief utterances with word errors (paraphasia). Repetition of words is impaired but powers of comprehension are relatively preserved. This is known as **Broca's aphasia**. There is also impairment of reading and writing (**alexia** and **agraphia**).

hemisphere (usually the left) lies the motor speech area, also known as **Broca's area** (Brodmann's areas 44 and 45). Broca's area has important interconnections with parts of the ipsilateral temporal, parietal and occipital lobes that are involved in language function.

The extensive regions of the cortex of the frontal lobe that lie anterior to premotor areas are referred to as **prefrontal cortex**. The prefrontal cortex has rich connections with parietal, temporal and occipital cortex through long association fibres running in the subcortical white matter. Subcortical afferents arise mainly in the mediodorsal and anterior nuclei of the thalamus. The prefrontal cortex has cognitive functions of a high order. These include intellectual, judgemental and predictive faculties and the planning of behaviour.

Parietal lobe

The parietal lobe lies behind the frontal lobe and is bounded posteriorly and inferiorly by the occipital and temporal lobes, respectively. The most anterior part of the parietal lobe is the postcentral gyrus, running parallel to the central sulcus (Figs 13.1, 13.2, 13.16). Functionally, this region is the **primary somatosensory cortex** (Brodmann's areas 1, 2 and 3). It is here that thalamocortical neurones terminate; these constitute the third and final relay in the chain from peripheral receptors for general sensation to a conscious level. The thalamic origin of these neurones is the ventral posterior nucleus, which in turn receives fibres of the medial lemniscus (fine touch and proprioception), spinal lemniscus (coarse touch and pressure), spinothalamic tracts (pain and temperature) and trigeminothalamic tracts (general sensation from the head). Within the somatosensory cortex, the contralateral half of the body is represented in an inverted, somatotopic pattern that resembles that in the primary motor cortex of the frontal lobe (Fig. 13.20).

Once again, the area of cortex devoted to a particular body part is disproportionate to the size of the latter; in the case of the sensory cortex it reflects rather the richness of sensory innervation. Therefore, the pharynx, tongue, face, lips and the palmar surface of the hands and digits are particularly well represented. Adjacent to the mouth area is a region where taste is perceived.

The surface of the parietal lobe posterior to the primary somatosensory cortex constitutes the parietal **association cortex**. The superior parietal lobule is responsible for the interpretation of general sensory information and for conscious awareness of the contralateral half of the body. Lesions here impair the interpretation and understanding of sensory input and may cause neglect of the opposite side of the body. The inferior parietal lobule interfaces between somatosensory cortex and the visual and auditory association cortices of the occipital and temporal lobes, respectively, and in the dominant hemisphere it contributes to language functions.

Parietal lobe lesions

Left parietal lobe lesions cause:

- Focal seizures – paroxysmal attacks of abnormal sensations, spreading down the contralateral side of the body (sensory seizures).
- Sensory/motor deficit – a contralateral hemisensory loss and inferior visual field loss.
- Psychological deficit – an inability to name objects (**anomia**) and a loss of literacy, with inability to read (**alexia**), to write (**agraphia**) and to calculate (**acalculia**).

Right parietal lobe lesions cause:

- Focal seizures – paroxysmal attacks of sensory disturbance affecting the contralateral side of the body (simple sensory seizures).
- Sensory/motor deficit – contralateral hemisensory loss and an inferior visual field loss.
- Psychological deficit – an inability to copy and construct designs because of spatial disorientation (**constructional apraxia**).

Temporal lobe

The lateral surface of the temporal lobe is divided into superior, middle and inferior temporal gyri, which run parallel to the lateral fissure. Within the superior temporal gyrus is located the **primary auditory cortex** (Brodmann's areas 41 and 42). More exactly, most of this functional zone lies in the superior bank of the gyrus, normally hidden within the lateral fissure. Its precise location is marked by the small transverse temporal gyri, or Heschl's convolutions (Fig. 13.17).

The primary auditory cortex is responsible for the conscious perception of sound and within it there is so-called 'tonotopical' representation of the cochlear duct. The primary auditory cortex receives input from the medial geniculate nucleus of the thalamus. The ascending acoustic projection undergoes partial decussation in the brain stem on its way to the medial geniculate nucleus (Ch. 10). At the cortical level, therefore, the organs of hearing are bilaterally represented so that unilateral lesions of the primary auditory cortex cause partial deafness in both ears. Auditory information is further processed and interpreted in the **auditory association cortex**, which lies surrounding and immediately posterior to the primary auditory cortex. In the dominant hemisphere, this region is also known as **Wernicke's area**. It is crucial for understanding of the spoken word and has important connections with other language areas of the brain.

The location of the cortical representation of the vestibular system is uncertain. There is evidence that it lies in the superior temporal gyrus anterior to the primary auditory cortex, or in the inferior parietal lobule.

The inferomedial part of the temporal lobe is curled inwards to form the **hippocampus**. This structure lies in the floor of the inferior horn of the lateral ventricle, deep to the parahippocampal gyrus (Figs 13.8–13.12, 13.16, see also Ch. 16). As part of the limbic system, the principal functions of the hippocampus are in relation to memory and the emotional aspects of behaviour. Close to the anterior end of the hippocampus and the temporal pole lies a mass of subcortical grey matter, the **amygdala**, which is also part of the limbic system. The amygdala and adjacent parts of the inferomedial temporal cortex receive fibres from the olfactory tract and are responsible for the conscious appreciation of the sense of smell. These connections receive further consideration in Chapter 16.

Left temporal lobe lesions

Left temporal lobe lesions cause:

- Focal seizures – paroxysmal attacks of unresponsiveness (**absences**), purposeless behaviour (**automatism**), olfactory and complex visual and auditory hallucinations, and disturbances of mood and memory (**déjà vu**). These attacks are referred to as complex partial seizures.
- Sensory/motor deficit – a contralateral superior visual field loss.
- Psychological deficit – speech that is fluent and rapid but contains word errors (paraphasia) and is incomprehensible. There is profound word-finding difficulty, impaired repetition of words, and profound loss of comprehension. This is known as **Wernicke's aphasia**.

Bilateral cortical disorders

Alzheimer's disease, a common degenerative disorder of the elderly, leads to atrophy of the temporal and parietal lobes and the limbic system (Fig. 13.21). It causes disorientation in space, and loss of language (**aphasia**) and memory (**amnesia**).

The common degenerative disorder of **frontotemporal dementia** leads to a total alteration of personality with loss of judgement, planning and insight, and the appearance of bizarre and uncharacteristic behaviour. Young people are affected.

Occipital lobe lesions

Occipital lobe lesions cause:

■ Focal seizures – paroxysmal visual hallucinations of a simple, unformed nature, such as lights and colours (simple partial seizures).
■ Sensory/motor deficit – a contralateral visual field loss (**contralateral homonymous hemianopia**).

Bilateral occipital lobe lesions lead to **cortical blindness**, of which the patient is unaware (**Anton's syndrome**). Bilateral occipitoparietal lesions can spare elementary vision but prevent the recognition and depiction of objects (**apperceptive visual agnosia**).

Language areas of the cerebral hemisphere

Certain higher cognitive functions are dealt with primarily, or even exclusively, by one of the cerebral hemispheres, which is then referred to as dominant for that function. In the great majority of people the left hemisphere is dominant for language and mathematical ability. The right hemisphere excels at spatial perception and musical proficiency. Cerebral dominance becomes established during the first few years after birth. During this formative period, both hemispheres exhibit linguistic ability and if one hemisphere sustains damage it may be compensated for by the plasticity of the developing brain and the child learns to speak normally. Later in life, this flexibility becomes greatly

Figure 13.21 Coronal section through the cerebral hemisphere of a patient dying with Alzheimer's disease, showing enlarged lateral ventricles and atrophic cortical gyri. (Courtesy of Professor D Mann, Clinical Neurosciences, Hope Hospital, University of Manchester, Manchester, UK.)

Occipital lobe

The occipital lobe lies behind the parietal and temporal lobes. On the medial surface of the hemisphere, the boundary with the parietal lobe is marked by the deep parieto-occipital sulcus. Also on the medial surface, the calcarine sulcus marks the location of the **primary visual cortex** (Brodmann's area 17; Fig. 13.16) which is responsible for visual perception. It occupies the gyri immediately above and below the calcarine sulcus, much of it being hidden in the depths of the sulci. This region receives fibres from the lateral geniculate nucleus of the thalamus by way of the optic radiation of the internal capsule. Each lateral half of the visual field is represented in the primary visual cortex of the contralateral hemisphere. The upper half of the visual field is represented below the calcarine sulcus, and the lower half is represented above the sulcus. The rest of the occipital lobe constitutes the **visual association cortex**. This region is concerned with the interpretation of visual images. Lesions of the primary visual cortex cause blindness in the corresponding part of the visual field, while damage to the visual association cortex causes deficits in visual interpretation and recognition. The visual system is considered in more detail in Chapter 15.

The cerebral cortex

■ The precentral gyrus is the primary motor region of the cerebral cortex and is located within the frontal lobe, immediately in front of the central sulcus. Anterior to this lie the premotor and supplementary motor cortices and, in the left hemisphere, Broca's (motor speech) area. The prefrontal cortex is concerned with complex cognitive functions.

■ The postcentral gyrus is the primary somatosensory region of the cerebral cortex and lies within the parietal lobe, immediately posterior to the central sulcus. It receives afferents from the ventral posterior nucleus of the thalamus, which is the site of termination of the spinothalamic tracts, trigeminothalamic tract and the medial lemniscus. Behind this region lies the sensory association cortex, which is responsible for the interpretation of general sensory information.

■ The temporal lobe lies beneath the lateral fissure. On the superior surface of the superior temporal gyrus, the transverse temporal gyri (Heschl's convolutions) mark the location of the primary auditory cortex, which receives input from the medial geniculate nucleus of the thalamus. Adjacent lies the auditory association cortex, which is responsible for the interpretation of auditory information and which, in the left hemisphere, constitutes Wernicke's area.

■ The occipital lobe makes up the posterior part of the hemisphere. On the medial surface, the calcarine sulcus indicates the location of the primary visual cortex, which receives afferents from the lateral geniculate nucleus of the thalamus. The rest of the occipital lobe is the visual association cortex, which is responsible for the interpretation of visual information.

diminished and damage to the dominant hemisphere often causes loss of speech in addition to the other deficits produced by hemispheric lesions.

The language areas of the brain are organised around the lateral fissure of the cerebral hemisphere. In the frontal lobe, Broca's area occupies the posterior part of the inferior frontal gyrus, adjacent to the motor cortical area for the head and neck. This region is concerned with expressive aspects of language (articulation). In the temporal lobe, the auditory association cortex, or Wernicke's area, is responsible for comprehension of the spoken word.

Nearby regions of the temporal lobe and parietal lobe, most notably the angular gyrus and supramarginal gyrus of the inferior parietal lobule, provide a functional interface between auditory and visual association areas important in naming, reading, writing and calculation.

White matter of the cerebral hemisphere

Beneath the cortical surface lies an extensive mass of nerve fibres, all of which have their origin or termination, and sometimes both, within the cortex. The fibres are classified into three types, depending upon their origin and destination:

1. **Association fibres**, which interconnect cortical sites lying within one cerebral hemisphere
2. **Commissural fibres**, which run from one cerebral hemisphere to the other, connecting functionally related structures
3. **Projection fibres**, which pass between the cerebral cortex and subcortical structures such as the thalamus, striatum, brain stem and spinal cord.

Association fibres

Some association fibres (Figs 13.22, 13.23) are short and link nearby areas of cortex by arching beneath adjacent cerebral sulci (U fibres). Other association fibres are longer and travel through the white matter to link distant areas of cerebral cortex. The primary sensory areas in the parietal, temporal and occipital lobes are linked by long association fibres to the association areas of the cerebral cortex. These, in turn, are connected to each other.

The large **superior longitudinal fasciculus** interconnects the frontal and occipital lobes. A subsidiary of this bundle, known as the **arcuate fasciculus**, links gyri in the frontal and temporal lobes that are important for language function.

Figure 13.22 **Coronal section of the cerebral hemisphere.** The diagram shows the location of the principal association, commissural and projection fibres.

Figure 13.23 **Principal association and commissural fibres of the cerebral hemisphere projected onto a median sagittal section.**

The **inferior longitudinal fasciculus** runs from the occipital to the temporal poles and contributes to the function of visual recognition.

The **uncinate fasciculus** connects the anterior and inferior parts of the frontal lobe with the temporal gyri, which are important structures in the regulation of behaviour. The **cingulum** lies within the cingulate gyrus and courses around the corpus callosum, connecting the frontal and parietal lobes with the parahippocampal and adjacent temporal gyri.

Associative agnosia

Cerebral damage, such as that caused by carbon monoxide poisoning, can destroy the inferior longitudinal fasciculus bilaterally. In such cases, the individual has intact elementary vision but cannot identify the nature of objects (**object agnosia**) or individual faces (**prosopagnosia**), although they can depict and match them.

Frontal pole

Anterior cerebral artery

Corpus callosum

Occipital pole

Figure 13.24 **Dissection of the brain from the superior aspect revealing the corpus callosum.**

Commissural fibres

The major interhemispheric commissural fibres are the corpus callosum, the anterior commissure and the hippocampal commissure (or commissure of the fornix) (Figs 13.22–13.26).

The **corpus callosum** spans the two cerebral hemispheres and connects corresponding regions of neocortex for all but the temporal fields (these have their own connection, the anterior commissure). The major parts of the corpus callosum, from rostral to caudal, are named the rostrum, genu, body and splenium. The corpus callosum is shorter rostrocaudally than is the hemisphere; as a result, callosal fibres linking the frontal or occipital poles curve forwards or backwards as the anterior and posterior forceps, respectively. The **splenium** interconnects the occipital cortices and, therefore, contributes to visual functions.

The **anterior commissure** runs transversely in front of the anterior column of the fornix and interconnects the inferior and middle temporal gyri and the olfactory regions on the two sides.

The **hippocampal commissure** consists of transverse fibres linking the posterior columns of the fornix on each side.

Damage to the corpus callosum

Patients with chronic epilepsy have undergone section of the corpus callosum to relieve their seizures. Such individuals betray few difficulties under normal circumstances. However, when these '**split-brain**' patients undergo psychological testing, the two halves of the brain appear to behave relatively autonomously. For example, visual information directed to the right, non-dominant, hemisphere alone does not evoke a verbal response; as a result, individuals cannot name objects or read words presented solely to the left visual field.

Destruction of the splenium of the corpus callosum by stroke or tumour leads to the posterior disconnection syndrome of **alexia without agraphia**. Such individuals speak and write without difficulty but cannot understand written material (alexia). Disconnection of visual processing in the right hemisphere from the verbal processing of the dominant left hemisphere is thought to explain the syndrome.

Corona radiata

Crus cerebri

Pontocerebellar fibres

Corticospinal fibres

Internal capsule

Figure 13.25 **Diffusion MRI tractography reconstruction of the projection fibres passing through the internal capsule.** Tractography measures the diffusion of water along axonal fibres and allows reconstruction of their trajectories in the living human brain. (Courtesy of Dr Marco Catani, Institute of Psychiatry, London, UK.)

Projection fibres

Projection fibres (Fig. 13.25) consist of afferent fibres conveying impulses to the cortex and efferent fibres conducting impulses away from it. The fibres projecting to and from the cerebral cortex are distributed radially as the corona radiata and then converge downwards towards the brain stem. The fibres become concentrated in a narrow area, called the **internal capsule**, between the thalamus and caudate nucleus medially, and the lentiform nucleus laterally. The internal capsule is angulated to form an anterior limb, genu, posterior limb and retrolenticular part (Fig. 13.26, see also Fig. 1.23).

The **anterior limb** contains connections between the mediodorsal nucleus of the thalamus and the prefrontal cortex, and also frontopontine fibres that project to the pontine nuclei in the basal portion of the pons.

The **posterior limb** contains corticobulbar and corticospinal motor fibres. Also within the posterior limb are thalamocortical projections passing from the ventral posterior nucleus to the primary somatosensory cortex, and from the ventral anterior and ventral lateral nuclei to motor regions of the frontal lobe.

Behind the posterior limb is a region referred to as the **retrolenticular** part of the internal capsule. This consists of fibres arising from the medial and lateral geniculate nuclei of the thalamus that pass to the auditory and visual cortices as the auditory and visual radiations, respectively. Visual thalamocortical fibres (also known as geniculocalcarine fibres) pass round the lateral ventricle and follow one of two courses to the visual cortex (Fig. 15.6). Those which represent the lower half of the visual field project to the upper part of the visual cortex (above the calcarine sulcus). They may be interrupted in their course by lesions of the parietal lobe. Fibres that represent the upper half of the visual field loop forwards over the inferior horn of the lateral ventricle (Meyer's loop) and may be damaged by lesions of the temporal lobe.

Rostrum of corpus callosum

Anterior limb of internal capsule

Genu of internal capsule

Posterior limb of internal capsule

Retrolenticular part of internal capsule

Splenium of corpus callosum

Figure 13.26 **Horizontal section of the cerebral hemisphere showing the parts of the internal capsule.**

White matter of the cerebral hemisphere

- Nerve fibres within the subcortical white matter are classified on the basis of their origin and termination.
- Association fibres link cortical regions within a single hemisphere. Important systems are: the superior longitudinal fasciculus, arcuate fasciculus, inferior longitudinal fasciculus and uncinate fasciculus.
- Commissural fibres pass between corresponding regions of the two hemispheres. The principal commissural system is the corpus callosum.

- Projection fibres run between the cerebral cortex and various subcortical structures. They pass through the corona radiata and the internal capsule. Particularly important fibres in this category are corticospinal, corticobulbar and thalamocortical projections.

Chapter 14
Corpus striatum

Within the cerebral hemisphere lie a number of nuclear masses. The most prominent of these are the **caudate nucleus**, **putamen** and **globus pallidus** which lie in close proximity to the internal capsule. They are collectively referred to as the **corpus striatum** or **basal ganglia** (Figs 14.1, 14.2; see also Figs 13.3–13.9, 13.14). The **amygdala**, which is located within the temporal lobe, near to the temporal pole, has a similar embryological derivation but is functionally quite different. It is part of the limbic system and is considered in Chapter 16.

The caudate nucleus, putamen and globus pallidus are anatomically and functionally related closely to each other and are principally involved in the control of posture and movement.

Abnormalities of posture and movement resulting from their dysfunction are commonly called basal ganglia disorders. The corpus striatum has important connections with other regions of the brain, particularly the cerebral cortex, the thalamus and subthalamic nucleus of the diencephalon, and the substantia nigra of the midbrain.

For gross anatomical purposes, the putamen and globus pallidus are sometimes together called the **lentiform (or lenticular) nucleus**. This is because they lie close together, forming an apparently single structure. The name means 'lentil-shaped', but a closer analogy would be a Brazil nut or the segment of an orange. The lentiform nucleus is three-sided, having a convex lateral surface and two other surfaces that converge to a medial apex which lies against the genu of the internal capsule. The term lentiform, or lenticular, is rather archaic and of limited use, although it is still retained in certain anatomical names (such as the retrolenticular part of the internal capsule).

On phylogenetic, connectional and functional grounds, however, the putamen is more closely allied to the caudate nucleus than to the globus pallidus. The globus pallidus is, in phylogenetic terms, the oldest part of the corpus striatum and is sometimes referred to as the **paleostriatum**. The abbreviation **pallidum** is more commonly used, particularly in composite terms for afferent and efferent connections, such as subthalamopallidal or pallidothalamic.

The caudate nucleus and putamen constitute the phylogenetically more recent **neostriatum** and are best regarded as a single entity. The two parts are almost (but not entirely) separated by the anterior limb of the internal capsule but their gross anatomical separation is not as significant as their neuronal and functional similarities. Together, they are commonly referred to simply as the **striatum**.

These rather confusing relationships are summarised in Figure 14.3.

Topographical anatomy of the corpus striatum

Striatum

The striatum (neostriatum) consists of the caudate nucleus and the putamen. Their combined three-dimensional shape is reminiscent of a tadpole, when viewed laterally (Fig. 14.4).

Putamen

The putamen lies lateral to the internal capsule and globus pallidus (Figs 14.1, 14.2; see also Figs 13.7, 13.8, 13.14). It is separated from the globus pallidus by a thin lamina of nerve fibres, the lateral medullary lamina. Lateral to the putamen lies more white matter, sandwiched within which lies a thin sheet of grey matter, known as the claustrum. This separates the white matter into two layers, the external capsule and the extreme capsule (Fig. 14.1). Lateral to the extreme capsule lies the cortex of the insula, deep within the lateral fissure of the hemisphere.

Caudate nucleus

The caudate nucleus consists of a large head and a tapering, curved tail. The head of the caudate is almost completely separated from the putamen by the internal capsule. At its rostral extremity, however, it is continuous with the putamen through and beneath the anterior limb of the internal capsule (Fig. 14.4, see also Figs 13.4–13.6). At this anterior level, the most ventral portion of the striatum is known as the **nucleus accumbens**, which has connections with the limbic system. The head of the caudate nucleus forms a prominent bulge in the lateral wall of the anterior horn of the lateral ventricle (Fig. 14.1, see also Figs 13.3–13.7). The tail of the caudate passes posteriorly, gradually tapering as it does so and, following the curvature of the ventricle, descends into the temporal lobe where it lies in the roof of the inferior horn (Fig. 14.4, see also Figs 13.9–13.12).

Figure 14.1 **Horizontal section of the brain showing the relationships of the corpus striatum.** Mulligan's stain has been used to increase the contrast between cell-rich areas (blue) and white matter.

Figure 14.2 **Coronal section of the brain showing the relationships of the corpus striatum.** Mulligan's stain (see legend to Fig. 14.1).

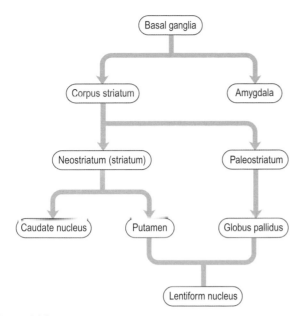

Figure 14.3 **Relationships of the nuclear masses within the cerebral hemisphere.**

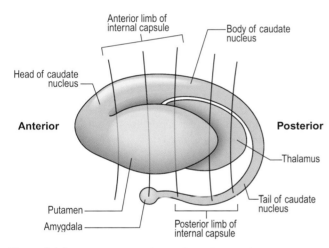

Figure 14.4 **Lateral aspect of the left caudate nucleus, putamen, amygdala and thalamus.** The globus pallidus is obscured by the putamen. The course of the internal capsule is shown in red. The putamen and the head of the caudate nucleus are separated by the anterior limb of the internal capsule, except at their most rostral extent where the two are in continuity. The posterior limb of the internal capsule separates the globus pallidus and putamen from the thalamus.

Globus pallidus

The globus pallidus lies medial to the putamen, separated from it by the lateral medullary lamina. Its medial apex nestles into the lateral concavity of the internal capsule (Fig. 14.1). The globus pallidus consists of two divisions, referred to as the external (or lateral) and the internal (or medial) segments. These are separated by a thin sheet of fibres, the medial medullary lamina (Fig. 14.1). The smaller medial segment shares many similarities, in terms of cytology and connections, with the pars reticulata of the substantia nigra in the midbrain. Although the two are separated by the internal capsule, these are best regarded as a single entity, in the functional sense.

Substantia innominata

The term substantia innominata refers to the basal part of the rostral forebrain that lies beneath the corpus striatum (see Fig. 14.7). This complex region contains several groups of neurones, one of them being the **nucleus basalis** (of Meynert), that project widely to the cerebral cortex and utilise acetylcholine as their neurotransmitter. These neurones undergo degeneration in Alzheimer's disease.

Functional anatomy of the corpus striatum

Connections of the striatum

The caudate nucleus and putamen, together commonly referred to as the striatum, are best considered as a single entity since they share common neuronal organisation, neurotransmitter systems and connections (Fig. 14.5). They are often regarded as the 'input' portions of the corpus striatum, since the majority of afferents from other parts of the brain end here rather than in the globus pallidus.

Striatal afferents

Afferents to the striatum come from three principal sources: the cerebral cortex, the thalamus and the substantia nigra.

Corticostriatal fibres originate from widespread regions of the cerebral cortex, predominantly, but not exclusively, of the ipsilateral side. Fibres from the frontal and parietal lobes predominate. Motor regions of the frontal lobe project mainly to the putamen, where the body is represented in an inverted, approximately somatotopic fashion. More anterior regions of the frontal lobe, and other association cortices, project mainly to the caudate nucleus. For these reasons, the putamen is considered to be the most overtly motor part of the striatum, the caudate nucleus having more associative functions. Corticostriatal fibres are excitatory to striatal neurones and use glutamic acid as their transmitter.

The **thalamostriatal projection** comes from the intralaminar nuclei (centromedian and parafascicular nuclei) of the ipsilateral thalamus.

The **nigrostriatal projection** originates from the **pars compacta** of the ipsilateral **substantia nigra** of the midbrain tegmentum. The transmitter used by this pathway

Figure 14.5 Schematic diagram illustrating the principal connections of the corpus striatum and related nuclei. Afferents to the striatum from the intralaminar thalamic nuclei and raphe nuclei have been omitted. For the sake of clarity, all efferents from the basal ganglia system are shown to originate from the medial segment of the globus pallidus, those from the pars reticulata of the substantia nigra being omitted. Similarly, efferents from the striatum are shown to originate only from the putamen and not from the caudate nucleus.

is the monoamine dopamine, which has both excitatory and inhibitory effects upon striatal neurones. The neurones of the pars compacta contain the dark pigment neuromelanin (Fig. 14.6), which is produced as a by-product of dopamine synthesis. The most rostral and ventral portion of the striatum, the nucleus accumbens, receives its dopaminergic input from the ventral tegmental area, which lies medial to the substantia nigra. This projection is known as the mesostriatal pathway. Other afferents to the striatum include a projection from the brain stem **raphe nuclei**, utilising serotonin as its transmitter.

Striatal efferents

The efferent projections of the striatum are directed principally to the two segments of the globus pallidus and to the pars reticulata of the substantia nigra (**striatopallidal** and **striatonigral fibres**, respectively). The cells of origin are so-called medium spiny neurones, which make up the vast majority of striatal nerve cells. Generally speaking, although there is some collateralisation, separate populations of neurones project to each of the three output targets. These projections are inhibitory upon pallidal and nigral neurones and utilise GABA as their primary transmitter. In addition, a number of neuropeptides are co-localised in these efferent neurones. The cells that project to the internal segment of the globus pallidus and the substantia nigra contain both **substance P** and **dynorphin**. The projection to the external segment of the globus pallidus contains **met-enkephalin**.

Figure 14.6 Transverse section through the midbrain showing the substantia nigra.

Connections of the striatum

- The caudate nucleus and putamen are the 'input' regions of the corpus striatum.
- They receive afferents from the cerebral cortex, intralaminar thalamic nuclei and the pars compacta of the substantia nigra.
- Efferent fibres are directed to the globus pallidus and the pars reticulata of the substantia nigra.

Connections of the globus pallidus

The two segments of the globus pallidus have similar afferent connections but substantially different efferent projections. The internal segment of the globus pallidus is very similar in structure and function to the pars reticulata of the substantia nigra, from which it is separated by the internal capsule. Together, the internal pallidum and pars reticulata of the substantia nigra are regarded as the 'output' portion of the basal ganglia, since they are the origin of the majority of basal ganglia efferent fibres that project to other levels of the neuraxis.

Pallidal afferents

Pallidal afferents arise principally from the striatum and from the subthalamic nucleus. Striatopallidal fibres are of two types, as previously noted, originating from different populations of striatal medium spiny neurones. Both utilise GABA as their primary transmitter. In addition, each contains characteristic peptide co-transmitters; fibres projecting to the external pallidal segment contain enkephalin, while those projecting to the internal pallidum contain substance P and dynorphin.

The **subthalamopallidal projection** originates in the subthalamic nucleus of the caudal diencephalon (Figs 14.7, 14.8). This small structure is located beneath the thalamus, lying against the medial border of the internal capsule. In coronal sections, it has the appearance of a biconvex lens. Subthalamopallidal fibres pass laterally through the internal capsule, contributing to a fibre system known as the **subthalamic fasciculus** (Fig. 14.8), and terminate in both segments of the globus pallidus, although termination is more dense in the internal segment.

The subthalamopallidal pathway is excitatory to pallidal neurones, using glutamic acid as its transmitter. The subthalamic nucleus also sends similar fibres to the pars reticulata of the substantia nigra, the other 'output' part of the basal ganglia system. The subthalamopallidal and subthalamonigral pathways have a pivotal role in the normal function of the basal ganglia and in the pathophysiology of basal ganglia disorders.

Figure 14.7 **Coronal sections through the corpus striatum and diencephalon.** Loyez method for myelin. (Sections courtesy of the National Museum of Health and Medicine, Armed Forces Institute of Pathology, Washington, DC, USA).

Figure 14.8 **Coronal section through the corpus striatum and diencephalon illustrating the efferent projections of the globus pallidus.**

Pallidal efferents

The two pallidal segments have different efferent projections. The external segment projects principally to the subthalamic nucleus. Pallidosubthalamic fibres pass medially through the internal capsule in the subthalamic fasciculus. This projection is inhibitory and uses GABA as its transmitter. The internal segment of the globus pallidus, together with the pars reticulata of the substantia nigra, projects primarily to the thalamus (ventral lateral, ventral anterior and centromedian nuclei), with a smaller projection to the brain stem tegmentum. These output neurones are all inhibitory and utilise GABA as their transmitter.

Pallidothalamic fibres take one of two routes to reach their target (Fig. 14.8). Some fibres pass round the anterior margin of the internal capsule as the **ansa lenticularis**, while others pass through the internal capsule as the **lenticular fasciculus**. The fibres continue to course medially and then loop dorsally and laterally as the **thalamic fasciculus** to enter the thalamus from its ventral aspect. In following this trajectory, pallidothalamic fibres circumnavigate a cellular region of the subthalamus known as the **zona incerta**, which lies between the thalamus and the subthalamic nucleus.

Pallidothalamic fibres constitute the main outflow from the basal ganglia. Their thalamic target nuclei (ventral anterior and ventral lateral), in turn, project excitatory, glutamatergic, fibres to the motor regions of the frontal lobe, principally the primary motor and supplementary motor cortices. A smaller contingent of medial pallidal efferent fibres passes caudally to terminate in the brain stem tegmentum in the **nucleus tegmenti pedunculopontinus (pedunculopontine nucleus)**, which lies at the boundary between midbrain and pons, surrounding the superior cerebellar peduncle (Fig. 14.5, see also Fig. 13.12). This region has been termed the **mesencephalic locomotor region** in lower mammals, since it is involved in the regulation of quadrupedal progression.

The pars reticulata of the substantia nigra is regarded as a homologue of the internal segment of the globus pallidus and, thus, has a similar status as the origin of basal ganglia output neurones. Like the internal pallidum, the pars reticulata receives fibres from the striatum and the subthalamic nucleus. The projection from the striatum is somatotopically organised, both in the pallidum and nigra, such that pallidal neurones are associated primarily with limb movements, whereas nigral cells control the axial musculature, including the extraocular muscles. As already noted, efferents from the internal pallidum project to the ventral anterior, ventral lateral and centromedian thalamic nuclei and to the pedunculopontine nucleus. Efferents of the pars reticulata of the substantia nigra also pass to a subregion of the ventral lateral thalamus, to the superior colliculus and to the brain stem reticular formation (including the pedunculopontine nucleus).

Connections of the globus pallidus

- The globus pallidus consists of two segments: external and internal.
- Both pallidal segments receive afferent fibres from the striatum and the subthalamic nucleus.
- The external pallidal segment projects to the subthalamic nucleus.
- The internal pallidal segment is homologous to the pars reticulata of the substantia nigra; the two structures are the 'output' regions of the basal ganglia.
- The internal pallidal segment projects to the thalamus (ventral anterior, ventral lateral and centromedian nuclei) and brain stem (pedunculopontine nucleus).

Normal functions of the basal ganglia

The basal ganglia are sometimes referred to as components of the so-called 'extrapyramidal motor system'. This term was coined to distinguish the symptoms seen clinically in diseases of the basal ganglia and related structures such as the substantia nigra and subthalamic nucleus, from the symptoms observed following stroke in the internal capsule, the latter being thought to be caused by destruction of the pyramidal tract. As understanding of the functional anatomy of the motor system has increased, it has become apparent both that the pyramidal and extrapyramidal systems are intimately related rather than separate, and also that so-called pyramidal signs are not all attributable to dysfunction of the pyramidal tract itself. The term extrapyramidal is, therefore, somewhat outdated but is still in widespread use.

Current concepts of the role of the basal ganglia consider that their function is to facilitate behaviour and movements that are required and appropriate in any particular context and to inhibit unwanted or inappropriate movements. How this might be achieved can be explained with reference to the internal connections of the basal ganglia (Fig. 14.5).

When a movement is initiated from the cerebral cortex, impulses discharge not only through corticospinal and corticobulbar pathways but also through the corticostriatal projection to the neostriatum. These glutamatergic fibres cause excitation of striatal medium spiny neurones. The striatum has two routes by which it is able to control the activity of basal ganglia output neurones in the internal segment of the globus pallidus and the pars reticulata of the substantia nigra. The first of these is the so-called 'direct pathway', consisting of striatopallidal and striatonigral neurones which directly inhibit internal pallidal or pars reticulata neurones. This mechanism has been shown to operate in experimental electrophysiological studies in primates, where basal ganglia output neurones associated with a particular body part or muscle group show a pause in their action potential discharge during movement of that region. This has been shown in the internal pallidum for limb movements and in the substantia nigra, pars reticulata for eye movements. Since internal pallidal and pars reticulata output neurones are themselves inhibitory, this leads to disinhibition of target neurones, including those of the motor thalamus. The resulting increase in the activity of thalamic neurones causes excitation of the cells of the cerebral cortex. The effect of activation of the direct pathway is, therefore, to support or facilitate ongoing movements, through this positive feedback to the cortex.

The second route by which striatal neurones can influence the output of the basal ganglia is the so-called 'indirect pathway', via the subthalamic nucleus. Efferents from the striatum terminate in the external pallidal segment and their activation induces inhibition of external pallidal neurones. The principal efferent projection of the external pallidum is to the subthalamic nucleus which, therefore, becomes disinhibited. The resultant increase in discharge of subthalamic neurones causes activation of internal pallidal and nigral neurones and, in turn, inhibition of thalamic and cortical cells. This has the effect of inhibiting unwanted movements.

Pathophysiology of basal ganglia disorders

Studies on the post-mortem brains of patients with **Parkinson's disease** and experimental animal studies have provided insight into the pathophysiological mechanisms that underlie the appearance of parkinsonian symptoms (Fig. 14.9). Normally, dopamine appears to exert an

Figure 14.9 **Schematic diagram illustrating how activities in basal ganglia and related nuclei become disordered in Parkinson's disease and chorea.** Overactive pathways are shown by solid lines; underactive pathways are shown by interrupted lines. For identification of structures, see Fig. 14.5.

Parkinson's disease | Chorea

excitatory influence upon striatal neurones of the 'direct' projection to the internal pallidal segment, and an inhibitory effect upon neurones of the 'indirect' pathway that projects to the external pallidal segment. Loss of striatal dopamine, therefore, causes abnormal underactivity of the direct pathway and disinhibition of internal pallidal neurones. Simultaneously, overactivity of the indirect projection leads to inhibition of external pallidal neurones, disinhibition of the subthalamic nucleus, and thus excessive excitatory drive of internal pallidal cells. Changes in both the direct and indirect pathways, thus, compound to exacerbate the abnormal overactivity of internal pallidal output cells, inducing akinesia.

The archetypal basal ganglia disease in which excessive, unwanted, abnormal movements (dyskinesias) occur is **Huntington's disease** (Huntington's chorea). Within the striatum, there is particular attrition of the cells that project to the external segment of the globus pallidus (the 'indirect' projection), at least early on in the condition. This leads to disinhibition of external pallidal neurones and inhibition of

the subthalamic nucleus. Internal pallidal neurones, therefore, become abnormally underactive and unwanted, involuntary movements ensue. Similar abnormal movements (chorea) occur as a complication of the long-term treatment of Parkinson's disease with L-DOPA. The underlying neural mechanism is similar but, in this case, there is both relative underactivity of the indirect pathway and overactivity of the direct pathway (Fig. 14.9).

Involuntary movement disorders

Unilateral basal ganglia lesions produce their effects on the contralateral side of the body, as is the case with cerebral hemisphere lesions, but distinct from cerebellar disorders. Basal ganglia dysfunction does not cause paralysis, sensory loss or ataxia, but leads to **abnormal motor control**, **alterations in muscular tone** and the emergence of abnormal, involuntary movements, or **dyskinesias**.

Abnormal motor control may consist of slowness of movement (**bradykinesia**) or poverty of movement (**hypokinesia, akinesia**). The initiation, sequencing and cessation of movement are disrupted. Normal posture cannot be maintained and 'associated' limb movements are lost, e.g. arm swinging when walking.

Tone may be increased throughout the range of passive movement (**rigidity**) and the hypertonia may be continuous (plastic) or discontinuous ('cogwheel'). Alternatively, **hypotonia** may occur.

Dyskinesias may be manifest in various ways and describe the abnormal movements, not the underlying disease. **Chorea** is a sequence of rapid, asymmetrical, and fragmented (quasi-purposeful) movements usually affecting the distal limb musculature. **Athetosis** consists of slow, sinuous, writhing movements. Sometimes movements share more than one characteristic; hence the term **choreo-athetosis**. **Dystonia** refers to sustained muscular contractions that give rise to abnormal postures or contortions. **Tremor** is a to-and-fro, sinusoidal movement that may be maximal at rest (resting tremor) or on action (action or postural tremor).

Tics are stereotyped movements, often highly characteristic of the individual, sometimes multiple and frequently influenced by emotional stress.

Myoclonus describes sudden, shock-like movements which are usually bilateral and especially affect the upper limbs.

Basal ganglia diseases

Parkinson's disease is a chronic neurodegenerative disease, usually occurring in the elderly. It is usually of unknown cause (idiopathic) although there are genetically determined forms which may be inherited. It is characterised by akinesia, a flexed posture, rigidity and a resting tremor. The pathological hallmark of Parkinson's disease is degeneration of the dopaminergic neurones of the pars compacta of the substantia nigra (Fig. 14.10), and depletion of striatal dopamine levels (Fig. 14.11). The most effective medical treatment currently available for the condition is administration of levodopa (L-DOPA), the immediate metabolic precursor of dopamine; dopamine receptor agonists may also be used. Levodopa is converted to dopamine and restores normal striatal function, a strategy that can often be used to minimise symptoms for many years. When drug therapy fails, neurosurgical ablation or electrical stimulation of the subthalamic nucleus or the internal segment of the globus pallidus can help the patient.

Huntington's disease is a chronic degenerative disease inherited in an autosomal dominant manner and characterised by chorea and progressive dementia. Pathologically, there is progressive degeneration of the striatum and cerebral cortex. **Hepatolenticular degeneration** (**Wilson's disease**) is an inherited disorder (autosomal recessive) of copper metabolism. Basal ganglia changes lead to choreo-athetosis and progressive dementia in childhood and youth. **Sydenham's chorea** is now rare but was formerly a common manifestation of rheumatic fever in young females, causing abnormal behaviour and generalised chorea (**St Vitus' dance**).

Levodopa-induced dyskinesia is a complication of the long-term treatment of Parkinson's disease with levodopa, and **tardive dyskinesia** is a long-term complication of the treatment of schizophrenia with neuroleptic drugs. **Hemiballism** is a rare condition characterised by violent choreiform movements of the limbs on one side of the body. It is caused by a lesion, usually of cerebrovascular origin, of the contralateral subthalamic nucleus. **Dystonia** may arise as an inherited disorder in children and is usually generalised. In adults, focal or segmental dystonias affect the arm and hand (writer's cramp), leg, neck (torticollis) or face and mouth (orofacial dyskinesia).

Figure 14.10 **Approximately transverse sections through the lateral half of the midbrain, showing degeneration and depigmentation of the substantia nigra, pars compacta in Parkinson's disease.** (Courtesy of Professor D Mann, Clinical Neurosciences, Hope Hospital, University of Manchester, Manchester, UK.)

Figure 14.11 **Positron emission tomography (PET) scans, representing horizontal sections through the brain at the level of the striatum.** Anterior is towards the top in each case. The top scans are from a normal individual and the bottom ones from a patient with Parkinson's disease. The scans on the left were made using the tracer [^{18}F]-dopa. This is taken up by intact dopaminergic nerve terminals and, therefore, acts as an index of the integrity of the nigrostriatal pathway. There is reduced labelling in the striatum of the parkinsonian patient. The scans on the right were made using the tracer [^{11}C]-raclopride. This binds to dopamine receptors located on striatal neurones that receive input from the nigrostriatal pathway. These receptors remain intact in the parkinsonian patient. (Courtesy of Professor D J Brooks, Hartnett Professor of Neurology, Imperial College, London, UK.)

Basal ganglia function

- The basal ganglia historically were referred to as parts of the extrapyramidal motor system to distinguish basal ganglia disorders from those of the pyramidal tract. However, both systems are intimately related.
- The basal ganglia facilitate purposeful behaviour and movement via the 'direct pathway' and inhibit unwanted movements via the 'indirect pathway'.
- Lesions of the basal ganglia produce effects on the contralateral side of the body.
- Diseases of the basal ganglia are typified by Parkinson's disease, in which there is poverty of movement, and Huntington's disease, which is associated with dyskinesias.

Chapter 15
Visual system

Vision is the most highly developed and versatile of all the sensory modalities and, arguably, the one on which humans are most dependent. The optic nerve and retina develop from the prosencephalic primary brain vesicle and, therefore, are regarded as an outgrowth of the brain itself. Vision commences with the formation of an image of the external world on the photoreceptive **retina**. The retina encodes visual information in the discharge of neurones that project to the brain through the **optic nerve**. Fibres of the optic nerve undergo hemidecussation in the **optic chiasma** and project to the lateral geniculate nucleus of the thalamus. Thalamocortical neurones in turn project to the primary visual cortex, in the occipital lobe of the cerebral hemisphere, where visual perception occurs.

The eye

The eyeball, or globe, is approximately spherical in shape (Fig. 15.1). Near its posterior pole emerges the optic nerve. The eyeball may be considered to consist of three concentric layers of tissue, the outermost of which is tough, fibrous and protective. Over most of the globe it forms an opaque white coat, the **sclera**, to which are attached the extraocular muscles that move the eyeball. Over the anterior pole of the globe it forms the transparent **cornea**, through which light enters the eye.

Near to the anterior margin of the sclera, two rings of smooth muscle extend into the lumen of the eyeball (Fig. 15.2). The most anterior of these is the **iris**, which has a central aperture, the **pupil**, through which light is admitted to the posterior part of the eye. Some of the muscle fibres of the iris are arranged in a circular fashion, while others are oriented radially. They are under the control of the autonomic nervous system. Circular fibres are innervated by postganglionic parasympathetic neurones, which act to constrict the pupil and reduce the amount of light falling upon the retina (see p. 100). Radial fibres are innervated by postganglionic sympathetic neurones which dilate the pupil.

Behind the iris lies the **ciliary body** containing **ciliary muscle**, which receives innervation from the parasympathetic nervous system. The central aperture within the annulus of the ciliary body is occupied by the transparent, biconvex **lens**, which focuses light upon the retina. The lens is held in place by a **suspensory ligament** that is attached to the peripheral margin of the lens and to the ciliary body. Contraction of the ciliary muscle alters the shape and, therefore, the focusing power (focal length) of the lens, a process known as accommodation. The lens and suspensory ligament divide the lumen of the eyeball into an anterior and a posterior part. The anterior part, in front of the lens, contains a thin, watery fluid, **aqueous humour**, which is continuously secreted from the ciliary body. It is also reabsorbed into the ciliary body where it is drained by a small duct, the **canal of Schlemm**, through which it is returned to the venous system. The posterior part of the globe contains a gelatinous material known as **vitreous humour**. Behind the ciliary body, the inner surface of the sclera is lined by the **choroid**, the cells of which contain dark pigment that absorbs light and thus reduces reflection within the eye. Lining the inner surface of the choroid is the photoreceptive retina.

Light passes from objects in the field of vision (**visual field**), through the narrow aperture of the pupil to subtend an image upon the retina. An object in the visual field, upon which attention is focused, subtends an image that is centred near the posterior pole of the eye along the line of the **visual axis** (Fig. 15.1). At this point, which is known as the **fovea centralis**, and the surrounding 1 cm, which is known as the **macula lutea**, the retina is specially modified for maximal visual acuity (resolving power). The basic optical properties of the eye, which may be likened to those of a pinhole camera, dictate that the image so formed is inverted in both lateral and vertical dimensions (Fig. 15.3). Furthermore, objects that lie in the left half of the visual field form an image upon the nasal (right) half of the left retina and the temporal (right) half of the right retina, and *vice versa*. Medial to the macula is a region where retinal axons accumulate to leave the eye in the optic nerve. This is known as the **optic disc**. Photoreceptors are absent from this region, which is also, therefore, referred to as the **blind spot**.

Retina

The retina consists of a non-neural and a neural portion. The non-neural part is represented by the **pigment epithelium**, a single layer of light-absorbing, pigmented cells lying adjacent to the choroid (Fig. 15.4). The neural part of the retina contains photoreceptors and neurones as well as neuroglia and a rich capillary network. The photoreceptive cells lie deepest within the retina and interdigitate with the pigment epithelium. Light entering the eye, therefore, passes through, and is refracted and partially absorbed by, these additional elements before reaching the photoreceptors. By means of a series of photochemical reactions and physicochemical changes, retinal photoreceptors transduce light energy into electrical energy (changes in membrane potential). Retinal photoreceptors

Figure 15.1 **Schematic drawing of a horizontal section through the right eyeball.**

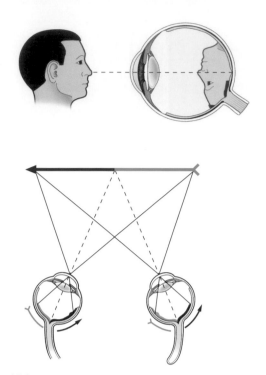

Figure 15.3 **The representation of the visual field upon the retinae.**

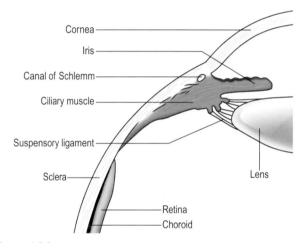

Figure 15.2 **Schematic drawing of the sclerocorneal junction of the eyeball.**

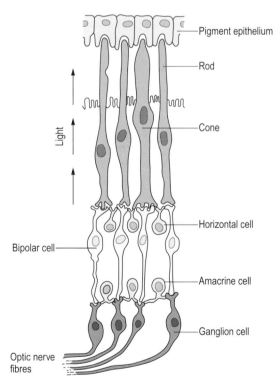

Figure 15.4 **Schematic drawing showing the cellular organisation of the retina.**

are of two types, **rods** and **cones**, of which the rods are about 20 times more numerous. These cells share many structural similarities but have important functional distinctions. Rods are exquisitely sensitive to light. They are particularly important for vision in dim lighting conditions. Cones are responsible for colour vision and, because of their arrangement and neuronal connections, they confer high visual acuity.

Rods and cones are heterogeneously distributed across the retina. Rods greatly predominate in the peripheral parts of the retina but their relative numbers decrease towards the macula, where cones are more abundant. At the fovea only cones are present. Furthermore, at the fovea the neurones and capillaries, through which light has to pass to reach the photoreceptors, are displaced so that the cones are directly exposed to light. This combination provides for maximal visual acuity.

In addition to photoreceptive cells, the retina contains the cell bodies of both the first- and second-order neurones of the central visual pathway (Fig. 15.4). The first-order neurone, or **bipolar cell**, lies entirely within the retina, while the axon of the second-order neurone, or **ganglion cell**, forms the optic nerve. Information is transferred from

photoreceptors to bipolar cells and then to ganglion cells, with greater convergence for rods than for cones. The retina also contains interneurones known as horizontal cells and amacrine cells. These modulate transmission between photoreceptors and bipolar cells, and between bipolar cells and ganglion cells, respectively.

The eye

- Objects in one lateral half of the visual field form images on the nasal half of the ipsilateral retina and the temporal half of the contralateral retina.
- The retina contains photoreceptors (rods and cones), first-order sensory neurones (bipolar cells) and second-order neurones (ganglion cells).
- The axons of retinal ganglion cells accumulate at the optic disc (blind spot) and pass into the optic nerve.

The central visual pathway

The axons of retinal ganglion cells assemble at the optic disc and pass into the optic nerve, which enters the cranial cavity through the optic canal. The two optic nerves converge to form the **optic chiasma** on the base of the brain (Fig. 15.5). The chiasma lies immediately rostral to the tuber cinereum of the hypothalamus and between the terminating internal carotid arteries. In the chiasma, axons derived from the nasal halves of the two retinae decussate and pass into the contralateral **optic tract**, while those from the temporal hemiretinae remain ipsilateral. The optic tracts diverge away from the chiasma and pass round the cerebral peduncle to terminate mainly in the lateral

geniculate nucleus (within the lateral geniculate body) of the thalamus. A relatively small number of fibres leave the optic nerve, before reaching the lateral geniculate nucleus, to terminate in the **pretectal area** and the superior colliculus. These fibres are involved in mediation of the pupillary light reflex (Ch. 10). From the lateral geniculate nucleus, third-order thalamocortical neurones project through the retrolenticular part of the internal capsule and form the **optic radiation**, which terminates in the primary visual cortex of the occipital lobe. The primary visual cortex is located predominantly on the medial surface of the hemisphere in the region above and below the calcarine sulcus. Surrounding this area, the rest of the occipital lobe constitutes the visual association cortex. It is concerned with interpretation of visual images, recognition, depth perception and colour vision.

There is a precise point-to-point relationship between the retina and the visual cortex. Because of the importance of the macula in vision, it is represented by disproportionately large volumes (relative to its size) of the lateral geniculate nucleus and the visual cortex. Within the visual cortex the macula is represented most posteriorly, in the region of the occipital pole.

As previously noted, objects in either half (left or right) of the visual field produce images upon the nasal hemiretina of the ipsilateral eye and the temporal hemiretina of the contralateral eye (Fig. 15.5). Each optic nerve, therefore, carries information concerning both halves of the visual field. Because of the decussation of fibres from the nasal hemiretinae at the optic chiasma, however, each optic tract, lateral geniculate nucleus and visual cortex receives information relating only to the contralateral half of the visual field. This combination of the images from both eyes is necessary for stereoscopic vision (depth perception). The upper half of the visual field forms images upon the lower halves of the retinae and the lower half of the visual field forms images upon the upper hemiretinae. As thalamocortical fibres leave the lateral geniculate nucleus they pass around the lateral ventricle, those representing the lower part of the visual field coursing superiorly to terminate in the visual cortex above the calcarine sulcus. Those which represent the upper part of the visual field sweep into the temporal lobe (**Meyer's loop**, Fig. 15.6) before terminating below the calcarine sulcus.

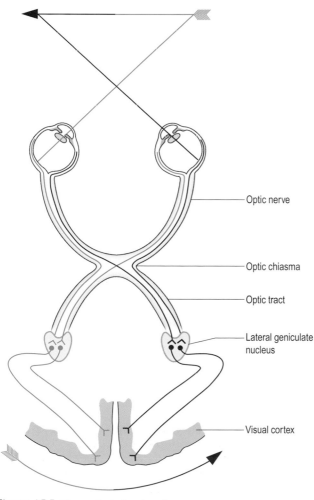

Optic nerve

Optic chiasma

Optic tract

Lateral geniculate nucleus

Visual cortex

Figure 15.5 **The central visual pathway.**

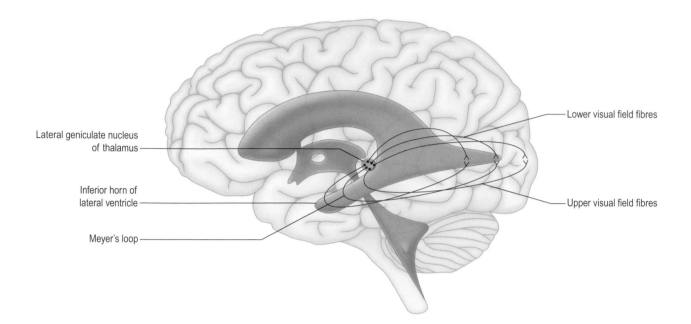

Figure 15.6 **The course taken by thalamocortical fibres projecting from the lateral geniculate nucleus to the primary visual cortex.**

The visual field can be considered (Fig. 15.7) as comprising four quadrants (left/right, upper/lower), each projecting to its own quadrant of the primary visual cortex (left/right hemispheres, above/below the calcarine sulcus). There is both lateral and vertical inversion in the projection of the visual field upon the visual cortex such that, for example, the upper left quadrant of the visual field is represented in the lower right quadrant of the visual cortex.

The central visual pathway

- At the optic chiasma, axons from the nasal halves of the two retinae decussate and pass into the contralateral optic tract.
- The optic tract contains axons that carry information relating to the contralateral half of the field of vision.
- Optic tract fibres end in the lateral geniculate nucleus of the thalamus.
- Third-order visual fibres from the lateral geniculate nucleus pass through the retrolenticular part of the internal capsule and the visual radiations to terminate in the primary visual cortex.
- The primary visual cortex is located above and below the calcarine sulcus of the occipital lobe.
- The rest of the occipital lobe constitutes the visual association area.

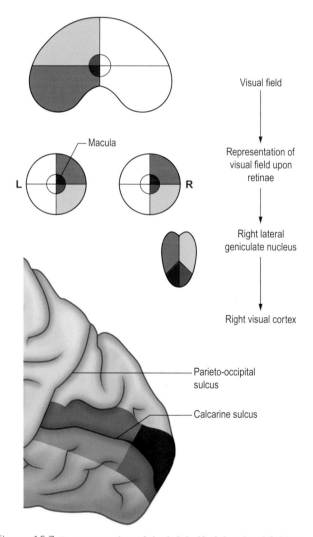

Figure 15.7 **Representation of the left half of the visual field at various levels in the visual pathway.**

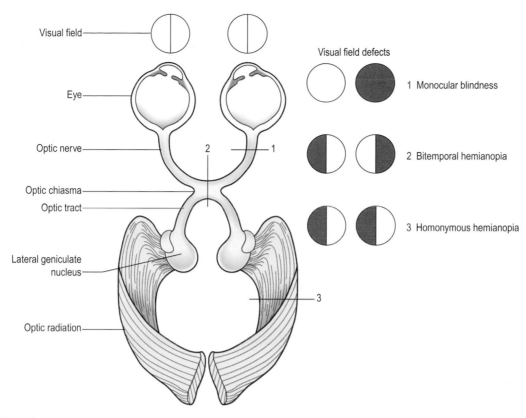

Figure 15.8 **Visual field deficits produced by lesions of the visual pathway.**

 Visual field deficits

Disease of the eyeball (cataract, intraocular haemorrhage, retinal detachment) and disease of the optic nerve (multiple sclerosis and optic nerve tumours) lead to loss of vision in the affected eye (**monocular blindness**). Compression of the optic chiasma by an adjacent pituitary tumour leads to **bitemporal hemianopia**. Vascular and neoplastic lesions of the optic tract, optic radiation or occipital cortex produce a contralateral **homonymous hemianopia** (Fig. 15.8).

Retinitis pigmentosa is an inherited metabolic disorder of the photoreceptor and retinal pigment epithelial cells. There is progressive night blindness, peripheral visual field constriction and pigmentation of the retina visible on ophthalmoscopy.

Chapter 16
Hypothalamus, limbic system and olfactory system

In order to survive, there must be continual adaptations to preserve the internal environment of the body (homeostasis). Interoceptor signals from the internal organs and body fluids initiate homeostatic responses; consequently, the internal physical and chemical environment remains balanced and stable. The hypothalamus is the structure responsible for this task.

Exteroceptive information from the outside world dictates behavioural responses, in order to achieve individual 'homeostasis' within the physical and social environment. Behaviour is relatively simple and stereotyped in lower animals and directed to satisfying the drives of thirst, hunger, sex and defence, in instinctive repertoires. The limbic system, which is strongly connected to the hypothalamus, is essential for this adaptive behaviour, which includes the ability to learn new responses based on previous experience (memory). The complex and non-stereotyped behaviour of humans is an attempt to preserve the individual within the physical landscape but also within a changing social environment (individual homeostasis). The association areas of the neocortex are capable of analysing exteroceptive information from the environment and other individuals, enabling adaptive personal and social responses. These phylogenetically more recent structures are partly connected to the limbic system.

As a result, the hypothalamus, limbic system and association neocortices act as interfaces in a hierarchical fashion between the internal structure of the individual and the environment. A reminder of this evolutionary ascent in humans is the olfactory system: vital for sensing the environment in lower animals, overwhelmed by visuospatial dominance in humans and intimately related to the limbic system.

Hypothalamus

The hypothalamus is able to integrate interoceptive signals from internal organs and fluid-filled cavities and make appropriate adjustments to the internal environment by virtue of its input and output systems.

The hypothalamic input is circulatory and neural in origin. The circulating blood provides physical (temperature, osmolality), chemical (blood glucose, acid–base state) and hormonal signals of the state of the body, its growth and development and its readiness for action (e.g. sex, suckling, defence etc). Neural signals come from two sources. First, the nucleus solitarius of the medulla projects to the hypothalamus and conveys information collected by the autonomic nervous system concerning the pressure within the smooth-muscled walls of organs (baroreceptors) and the chemical constituents of the fluid-filled cavities (chemoreceptors). Second, the state of neural arousal is communicated by two structures in the midbrain: the reticular formation via direct and indirect (via thalamus) routes, and the monoaminergic nuclei via the medial forebrain bundle.

The hypothalamus is capable of generating responses to these stimuli by circulatory and neural means. An intimate relationship with the pituitary gland and privileged access to its circulation (portal system) confers the role of 'orchestrator of the endocrine system' on the hypothalamus, as it directs hormonal synthesis and release. The neural output of the hypothalamus is two-fold. First, the autonomic nervous system projects to and controls internal organs, outside conscious control (and, hence, autonomous). Second, the hypothalamus is capable of initiating appropriate motor behavioural repertoires of an instinctive kind through its connections with the limbic system and limbic part of the corpus striatum (the nucleus accumbens). Its interconnections with the reticular formation also are capable of influencing the state of wakefulness and sleep.

The hypothalamus has the capability of influencing or overriding more complex adaptive behaviour because of its close links with two important structures: the limbic system and the association cortex of the frontal lobe (orbital part).

Topographical anatomy of the hypothalamus

The hypothalamus is the most ventral part of the diencephalon, lying beneath the thalamus and ventromedial to the subthalamus (Fig. 16.1). It forms the floor and the lower part of the lateral wall of the third ventricle, below the hypothalamic sulcus (see Fig. 12.2). On the base of the brain, parts of the hypothalamus can be seen occupying the small area circumscribed by the crura cerebri, optic chiasma and optic tracts (see Fig. 12.1). Between the rostral limits of the two crura cerebri, on either side of the midline, lie two distinct, rounded eminences, the **mammillary bodies**, which contain the **mammillary nuclei**. In the midline, immediately caudal to the optic chiasma, lies a small elevated area known as the **tuber cinereum**, from the apex of which extends the thin **infundibulum** (infundibular

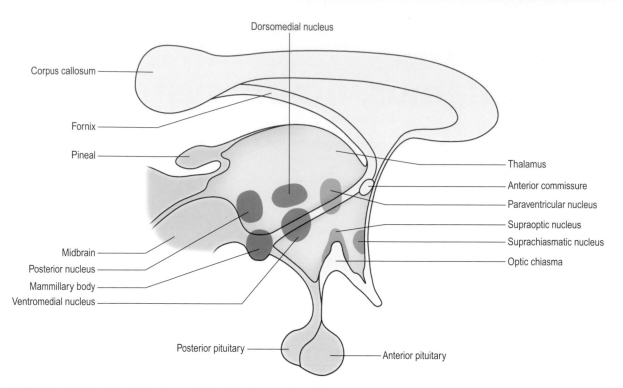

Figure 16.1 **A sagittal section of the diencephalon.** The diagram shows the medial aspect of the hypothalamus. The approximate location of some of the principal hypothalamic nuclei is shown.

Figure 16.2 **Supraoptic and paraventricular nuclei projecting to the posterior pituitary via the hypothalamohypophyseal tract.**

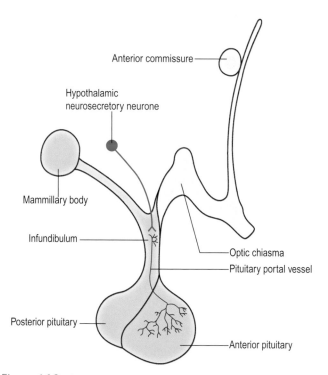

Figure 16.3 **Pituitary portal system linking anterior and posterior parts of the pituitary gland.**

process), or **pituitary stalk**. This is attached to the **pituitary gland** (**hypophysis**), a pea-sized structure which lies within the sella turcica of the sphenoid bone. The pituitary gland consists of two major, cytologically distinct, parts: the posterior pituitary or **neurohypophysis** and the anterior pituitary or **adenohypophysis** (Figs 16.2, 16.3). The posterior pituitary is a neuronal structure, being an expansion of the distal part of the infundibulum. The anterior pituitary is not neural in origin. The two parts are, however, closely linked by the **pituitary** (hypophyseal) **portal system** of vessels (Fig. 16.3), which are derived from the superior hypophyseal artery. Releasing factors, which

are synthesised in the hypothalamus, pass to the adenohypophysis through these vessels to control the release of anterior pituitary hormones.

Hypothalamic nuclei

The hypothalamus consists of many nuclear divisions, only some of which will be described (Fig. 16.1). The region lying medial and ventral to the structures of the subthalamus is known as the **lateral hypothalamus**. It is traversed longitudinally by many fibres, including the medial forebrain bundle. The lateral hypothalamic area is important in the control of food and water intake and is, in part, equivalent to the physiologically defined feeding centre. Lateral hypothalamic lesions cause aphagia and adipsia.

The medial region of the hypothalamus contains various nuclei, only some of which have well-defined functions. Anteriorly lie the supraoptic, paraventricular and suprachiasmatic nuclei. The supraoptic and paraventricular nuclei both produce systemically acting hormones, which are released from the posterior pituitary into the general circulation. The **supraoptic nucleus** produces vasopressin (antidiuretic hormone), which increases water reabsorption by the kidney. The **paraventricular nucleus** synthesises oxytocin. In the female, activation of the paraventricular nucleus, and release of hormone, is induced by suckling. This stimulates milk production by the mammary gland and causes contraction of uterine muscle.

The axons of cells in the supraoptic and paraventricular nuclei pass to the neurohypophysis in the hypothalamohypophyseal tract (Fig. 16.2). The neuroendocrine products are transported in this tract to the neurohypophysis, where they are released into the capillary bed and, thus, reach the general circulation.

The supraoptic nucleus contains osmosensitive neurones that are activated by changes in the osmolality of circulating blood. An increase in osmolality causes release of vasopressin. This acts upon the kidney tubules to increase water reabsorption, thus maintaining water homeostasis.

The hypothalamus also synthesises releasing factors and release-inhibiting factors, which control the release of hormones by the adenohypophysis. The adenohypophysis produces adrenocorticotropic hormone (ACTH), luteinising hormone (LH), follicle-stimulating hormone (FSH), thyroid-stimulating hormone (TSH), growth hormone and prolactin, which are released into the general circulation. The factors that control them are released from the terminals of hypothalamic neurones into the capillary bed of the pituitary portal system (Fig. 16.3). These vessels, which are intrinsic to the hypophyseal stalk, convey the released agents to the adenohypophysis, where they act upon the hormone-secreting cells. The synthesis of hypothalamic releasing factors is under feedback regulation by hormones produced by target organs.

Tumours of the hypothalamus and pituitary gland

Tumours and other diseases of the hypothalamus and associated pituitary gland lead to under- or overproduction of circulating hormones. These, in turn, produce disorders of growth (**dwarfism**, **gigantism** and **acromegaly**), sexual function (**precocious puberty**, **hypogonadism**), body water control (**diabetes insipidus** and **pathological drinking**), eating (**obesity** and **bulimia**) and adrenal cortical control (**Cushing's disease** and **adrenal insufficiency**). Since the pituitary gland is closely adjacent to the optic chiasma, tumours of the gland (**pituitary adenomas**) may lead to bitemporal visual field loss.

Hypothalamus

- The hypothalamus is part of the diencephalon; it is connected to the pituitary gland via the infundibulum.
- The hypothalamus has autonomic, neuroendocrine and limbic functions and is involved in the coordination of homeostatic mechanisms.
- The hypothalamus produces hormones that are released from the posterior pituitary and also releasing factors that control the release of hormones from the anterior pituitary.
- The supraoptic and paraventricular nuclei of the hypothalamus produce vasopressin and oxytocin, respectively.
- Vasopressin and oxytocin are transported to the posterior pituitary in the hypothalamohypophyseal tract.
- The anterior pituitary produces: adrenocorticotropic hormone, luteinising hormone, follicle-stimulating hormone, thyroid-stimulating hormone, growth hormone and prolactin. Factors that control their secretion are released into the pituitary portal system of the pituitary stalk and carried to the anterior pituitary.
- The lateral hypothalamus and the ventromedial nucleus regulate eating and drinking.

The **suprachiasmatic nucleus** is concerned with the control of diurnal rhythms and the sleep/waking cycle. It receives some afferent fibres directly from the retina.

More caudally, dorsomedial and ventromedial nuclei lie deep to the lateral wall of the third ventricle. The **ventromedial nucleus**, like the lateral hypothalamus, is concerned with the control of food and fluid intake. The ventromedial nucleus is equated with the physiologically defined satiety centre and lesions of this region cause abnormally increased food intake. In the most caudal part of the hypothalamus lie the posterior nucleus and the **medial mammillary nucleus**, the latter being located within the mammillary body. The mammillary body is part of the limbic system, receiving afferents from the hippocampus and projecting to the anterior nuclei of the thalamus and the brain stem.

The hypothalamus is the brain centre for regulation of the autonomic nervous system. Generally, activation of the posterior hypothalamic domain is associated with sympathetic responses, whereas activation of the anterior hypothalamus is associated with parasympathetic activity.

Limbic system

The limbic system earns its title from its position on the medial rim of the brain (*le grand lobe limbique*). It consists of a number of structures with complex and often looped connections that all ultimately project into the hypothalamus (Fig. 16.4). The powerful input to the limbic system from the neocortical association areas links complex 'goal-directed' behaviour to more primitive, instinctive behaviour and internal homeostasis in a cascade of neural connections (Figs 16.5, 16.6). In a simplified way, we may conceive of information from the outside world collected in modality-specific ways (e.g. vision, hearing and touch) and refined in the parieto-occipital association areas (perceptuospatial function). This information is then conveyed to the frontal association areas involved in planned behaviour (regulation) and also to the inferior temporal association areas, where information can reach supramodal status and meaning (semantic processing). Entry of information into the limbic system is either directly to the amygdala, or indirectly to the hippocampal formation, via the entorhinal area. The amygdala appears to provide an affective connotation to experience and especially that relevant to social stimuli. Perhaps affect is an evolutionary development from more primitive 'feelings', derived from the sensory autonomic input from bodily organs into the hypothalamus. The informational flow into the hippocampal formation permits a link to previous experience since the hippocampal formation is essential to remembering and learning (memory).

The limbic system is able to influence motor responses appropriate to its informational analyses, through projections to the nucleus accumbens, which forms part of the basal ganglia.

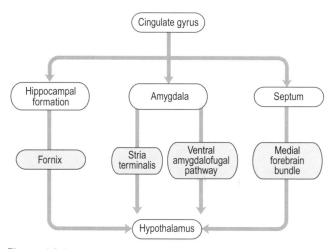

Figure 16.4 **The principal parts of the limbic system and their relationship with the hypothalamus.**

Amygdala

The amygdala lies near the temporal pole, between the inferior horn of the lateral ventricle and the lentiform complex (Fig. 16.7, see also Fig. 13.8). It receives afferents from the inferior temporal association cortex, the septum and the olfactory tract. In addition it receives catecholamine- and serotonin-containing projections from the brain stem in the medial forebrain bundle. The principal efferent projection from the amygdala is the stria terminalis, which runs in the wall of the lateral ventricle, following the curvature of the caudate nucleus, to terminate ultimately in the hypothalamus. The ventral amygdalofugal path also projects to the hypothalamus.

Septum

The septum, or septal region, lies beneath the rostral part of the corpus callosum (Fig. 16.7). It interconnects with the amygdala and projects to the hypothalamus via the medial forebrain bundle. The septum also connects to the monoaminergic nuclei in the brain stem. It does so via fibres that project to the **habenular nuclei** of the diencephalon and constitute the **stria medullaris thalami**. The habenular nuclei in turn project, via the fasciculus retroflexus, to the **interpeduncular nuclei**, which project to the brain stem as well as the hypothalamus. In this way, two major pathways link the septum, the hypothalamus and the monoaminergic nuclei of the brain stem.

Hippocampal formation

The hippocampal formation consists of the hippocampus itself, the dentate gyrus and parts of the parahippocampal gyrus. The **hippocampus** is formed by an infolding of the inferomedial part of the temporal lobe into the lateral ventricle, along the line of the choroid fissure (Fig. 16.8, see also Figs 13.8–13.12). The **dentate gyrus** lies between the parahippocampal gyrus and the hippocampus.

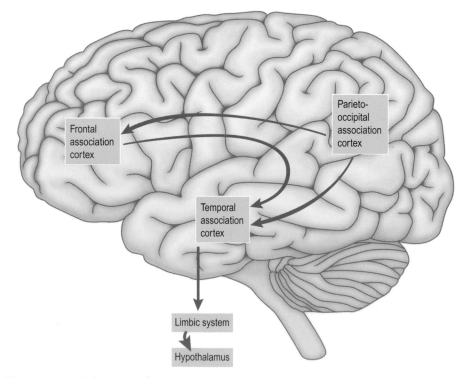

Figure 16.5 **The link between associative areas of neocortex, the limbic system and the hypothalamus.**

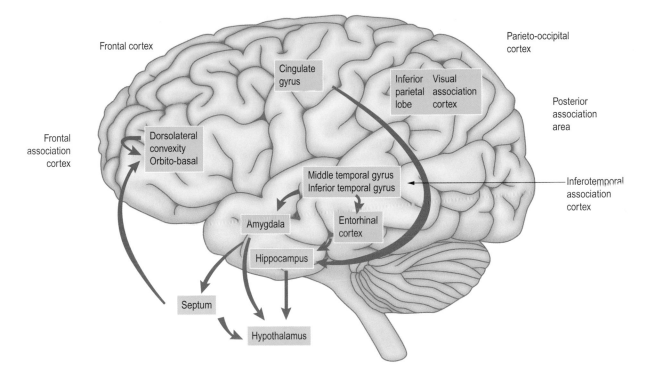

Figure 16.6 **The interconnections between associative neocortical regions and the component parts of the limbic system.**

Figure 16.7 **Coronal section of the brain showing the location of the amygdala and anterior commissure and their relationships with the basal ganglia.** Mulligan's stain (see Fig. 1.5).

Figure 16.8 **Transverse section through the hippocampus and inferior horn of the lateral ventricle.**

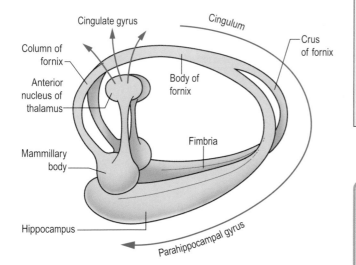

Figure 16.9 **The interconnection of limbic structures that constitute the Papez circuit.**

The hippocampal formation receives afferents principally from the inferior temporal cortex via the entorhinal area of the temporal lobe. It also receives fibres from the contralateral entorhinal area and hippocampus via the fornix system and hippocampal commissure. The principal efferent pathway from the hippocampus is the **fornix** (Figs 16.9–16.11, see also Figs 12.2, 13.2, 13.7–13.12). The fornix is a prominent C-shaped fascicle of fibres that links the hippocampus with the mammillary body of the hypothalamus. Efferent fibres converge on the ventricular surface of the hippocampus as the **fimbria**. This passes posteriorly and superiorly to become continuous with the

crus of the fornix, which then curves forward beneath the splenium of the corpus callosum (Fig. 16.12). The two crura unite in the midline, beneath the corpus callosum, to form the body of the fornix (Fig. 16.10); some fibres cross to the opposite side through the small hippocampal commissure. As it passes forwards beneath the corpus callosum, the body of the fornix divides into two columns. These curve downwards, forming the anterior border of the interventricular foramen, and enter the hypothalamus, where the majority of fibres terminate in the mammillary body. The mammillary body, in turn, projects to the anterior nuclear group of the thalamus via the mammillothalamic tract and to the brain stem via the mammillotegmental tract. The anterior nuclei of the thalamus have major connections with the cingulate gyrus.

Cingulate gyrus

The cingulate gyrus and the **parahippocampal gyrus** are in continuity with one another around the splenium of the corpus callosum (Fig. 13.16). The cingulate gyrus projects to the parahippocampal gyrus via the fibres of the cingulum (Ch. 13). The principal structures of the limbic system are thus linked by a series of connections, which constitute the **Papez circuit** (Figs 16.9, 16.10).

Limbic system

- The amygdala is located near to the temporal pole. It receives projections from the olfactory system and the temporal cortex, and has reciprocal connections with the septum.
- The hippocampal formation is made up of the hippocampus, dentate gyrus and parahippocampal gyrus of the temporal lobe. It receives fibres from the entorhinal cortex and projects via the fornix to the mammillary body of the hypothalamus.
- The principal components of the limbic system are interconnected in the Papez circuit.

Limbic lobe disorders

Alcohol abuse, in a setting of dietary deficiency of thiamine, leads to capillary haemorrhages in the upper brain stem and limbic structures. The patient falls into confusion and coma (**Wernicke's encephalopathy**). Partial recovery may occur, with failure to remember previous experience (retrograde amnesia) or to learn new facts (anterograde amnesia). This is known as **Korsakoff's psychosis**. A similar amnesic syndrome occurs when bilateral, surgical temporal lobectomy incorporates the hippocampal formations.

Temporal lobe or **complex partial seizures** arising close to the amygdala and hippocampi can lead to complex experiences of smell, mood and memory. The states of disordered thinking, hallucinations and strange or violent behaviour can mimic schizophrenia. Surgical ablation of the amygdala has eliminated uncontrollable rage reactions in some psychotic patients.

Figure 16.10 **Dissection of the medial aspect of the diencephalon to show the relationships of the fornix, mammillary body and mammillothalamic tract.**

Figure 16.11 **The Papez circuit projected onto the medial aspect of the cerebral hemisphere.**

Olfactory system

Olfactory receptors are specialised, ciliated nerve cells that lie in the olfactory epithelium of the nasal cavity. Their axons assemble into numerous small fascicles (the true olfactory nerves) that enter the cranial cavity through the foramina of the **cribriform plate** of the ethmoid bone (see Fig. 5.1) and then attach to the **olfactory bulb** on the inferior surface of the frontal lobe (Fig. 16.13, see also Fig. 10.1). Preliminary processing of olfactory information occurs within the olfactory bulb, which contains interneurones and large **mitral cells**; axons from the latter leave the bulb in the olfactory tract.

The olfactory tract passes backwards on the basal surface of the frontal lobe and, just before reaching the level of the optic chiasma, most olfactory tract fibres are deflected laterally, in the **lateral olfactory stria** (Fig. 16.13). These fibres pass into the depths of the lateral fissure, which they cross to reach the temporal lobe. They terminate mainly in the **primary olfactory cortex** of the **uncus** (Fig. 16.13, see also Fig. 13.2), on the inferomedial aspect of the temporal lobe, and in the subjacent amygdala. Adjacent to the uncus, the anterior part of the parahippocampal gyrus, or entorhinal area, constitutes the olfactory association cortex. The primary and association cortices are also collectively referred to as the pyriform cortex and are responsible for the appreciation of olfactory stimuli. The olfactory projection is unique among the sensory systems in that it consists of a sequence of only two neurones between the sensory receptors and cerebral cortex and does not project via the thalamus.

Head of caudate nucleus

Anterior horn of lateral ventricle

Crus of fornix

Thalamus

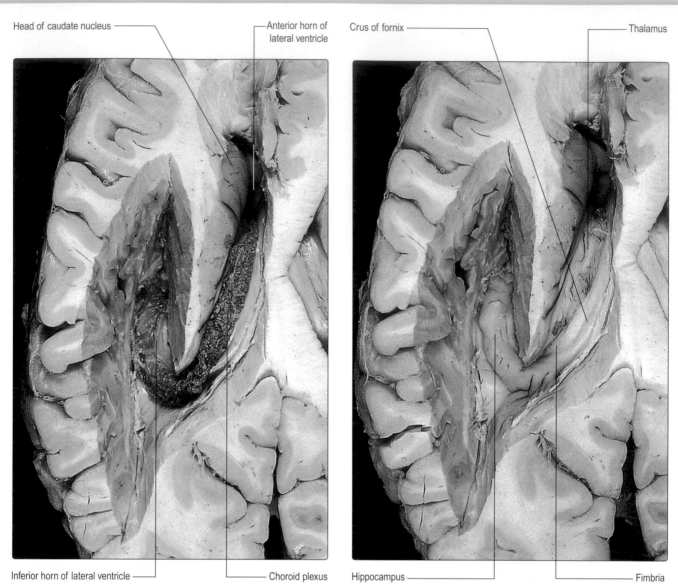

Inferior horn of lateral ventricle

Choroid plexus

Hippocampus

Fimbria

Figure 16.12 **The hippocampus–fimbria–fornix system.** The brain is viewed from above. The cerebral cortex and white matter, including the corpus callosum, have been removed to reveal the lateral ventricle and its contents. **(A)** Choroid plexus of lateral ventricle intact; **(B)** Choroid plexus removed.

Olfactory bulb

Olfactory tract

Frontal lobe

Lateral olfactory stria

Optic nerve

Anterior perforated substance

Optic tract

Mammillary body

Crus cerebri

Parahippocampal gyrus

Uncus

Posterior perforated substance

Pons

Figure 16.13 **Ventral surface of the brain.** The illustration shows the olfactory bulb and tract, the lateral olfactory stria and the primary olfactory area of the cerebral cortex (uncus).

Olfactory system

- Olfactory nerve fibres terminate in the olfactory bulb.
- Second-order fibres run in the olfactory tract and terminate in the primary olfactory cortex of the uncus in the temporal lobe.
- Adjacent to this, the anterior part of the parahippocampal gyrus, or entorhinal cortex, constitutes the olfactory association cortex.

Anosmia

Anosmia follows damage to the olfactory nerves. There is loss not only of the sense of smell but also of the flavour of foods. However, elementary aspects of taste, e.g. sweet, salt, bitter and sour, are preserved. Anosmia frequently follows head trauma and can occur when tumours of the meninges (**meningiomas**) invade the olfactory nerves.

Chapter 17
Problem-solving

Introduction

Neuroanatomy is primarily an anatomical rather than a clinical textbook. Neuroanatomy is, however, the foundation of clinical neurological diagnosis. This is because the clinical syndromes arising from lesions within the neuromuscular system are determined by the topographical location of the lesion, rather than by its cause. Thus, by combining knowledge of neuroanatomy with the practical skills of the clinical examination, the site of the lesion can be determined with great accuracy at the bedside and before the application of sophisticated investigations. Once the clinical syndrome is defined and the site of the lesion within the nervous system located, it is possible to infer the cause of the lesion by a careful consideration of the evolution of the patient's symptoms, obtained by clinical history-taking. The ultimate diagnosis is reached by applying appropriate investigations in order to clarify the site and cause of the lesion.

In order to exemplify this diagnostic process, a series of problem-solving tasks is presented. These provide sufficient information concerning the clinical neurological findings on examination to permit deduction of the site of the lesion within the neuromuscular system.

Throughout the text, simplified summaries of the major anatomical–clinical syndromes are presented diagrammatically, following the conventional neurological examination of cranial nerves, motor function, reflexes, sensation, coordination and mental state, described in textbooks of clinical methods. These figures follow a standard style exemplified by Figure 17.1.

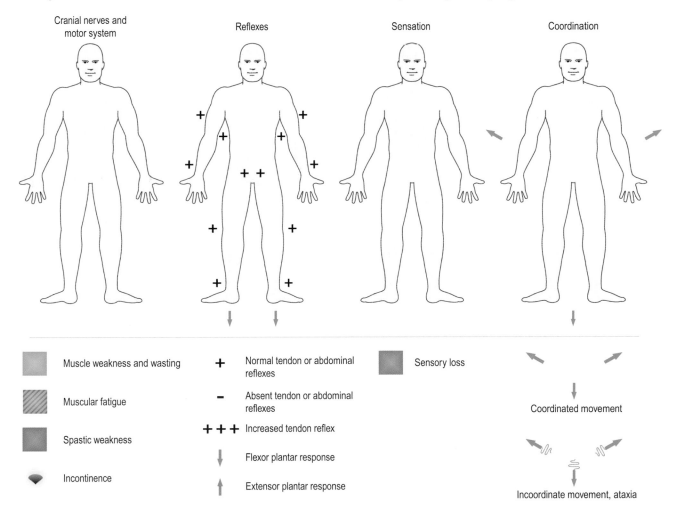

Figure 17.1 **Prototypical figure for illustration of major syndromes of the neuromuscular system.**

Problems

The figures from the foregoing text that summarise the major anatomical–clinical syndromes are reproduced below (Figs 17.2–17.13), with the omission of the small inset diagram that identifies the site of the lesion. In each case, the task is to study the findings of the clinical examination and thereby deduce the location of the lesion. The aetiology of the lesions can also be inferred from study of Figures 1.31–1.39 (Aetiology of neurological disease; Ch. 1) which link aetiologies to neuroanatomical sites.

Figure 17.2

Figure 17.3

Figure 17.4

Figure 17.5

Figure 17.6

Figure 17.7

Figure 17.8

Figure 17.9

Figure 17.10

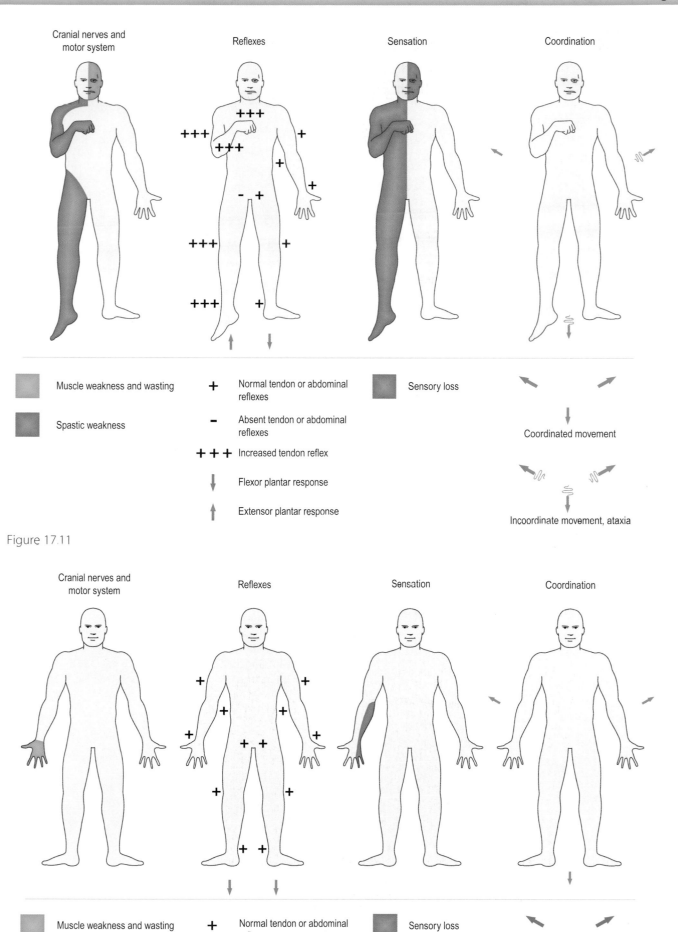

Cranial nerves and motor system Reflexes Sensation Coordination

⬛	Muscle weakness and wasting	
⬛	Spastic weakness	

+ Normal tendon or abdominal reflexes

− Absent tendon or abdominal reflexes

+ + + Increased tendon reflex

↓ Flexor plantar response

↑ Extensor plantar response

⬛ Sensory loss

Coordinated movement

Incoordinate movement, ataxia

Figure 17.11

Cranial nerves and motor system Reflexes Sensation Coordination

⬛	Muscle weakness and wasting	

+ Normal tendon or abdominal reflexes

↓ Flexor plantar response

⬛ Sensory loss

Coordinated movement

Figure 17.12

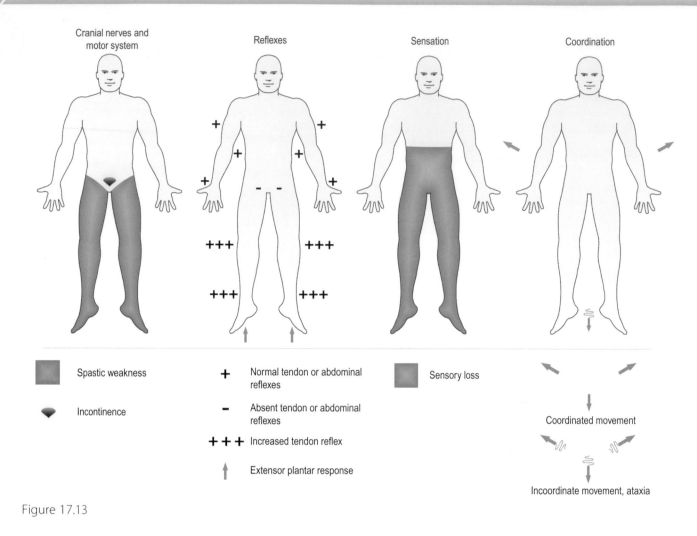

Cranial nerves and motor system

Reflexes

Sensation

Coordination

▨	Spastic weakness	**+**	Normal tendon or abdominal reflexes
◆	Incontinence	**–**	Absent tendon or abdominal reflexes
		+ + +	Increased tendon reflex
		↑	Extensor plantar response

▨ Sensory loss

Coordinated movement

Incoordinate movement, ataxia

Figure 17.13

Solutions to task

Figure 17.2: Upper cervical spinal cord lesion (see Fig. 8.21A).

Figure 17.3: Peripheral sensorimotor neuropathy (see Fig. 3.10).

Figure 17.4: Hemisection of the spinal cord (see Fig. 8.21E).

Figure 17.5: Myopathy (see Fig. 3.2).

Figure 17.6: Unilateral cerebral hemisphere lesion (see Fig. 13.19).

Figure 17.7: Myasthenia gravis (see Fig. 3.8).

Figure 17.8: Lower cervical spinal cord lesion (see Fig. 8.21B).

Figure 17.9: Spinal nerve root lesion (see Fig. 8.7).

Figure 17.10: Lumbar spinal cord lesion (see Fig. 8.21D).

Figure 17.11: Unilateral brain stem lesion (see Fig. 9.14).

Figure 17.12: Brachial plexus lesion (see Fig. 3.12).

Figure 17.13: Thoracic spinal cord lesion (see Fig. 8.21C).

Glossary

Acalculia – Inability to calculate

Accommodation – Act of refocusing the visual image

Acromegaly – Overgrowth of the skeleton and organs caused by excessive release of growth hormone from a pituitary tumour

Acuity – Resolving power

Action potential – Transient reversal of the resting potential that is propagated along the axon

Adenoma – Benign tumour

Adhesion – Scarring of tissues, fixing them together

Adipsia – Inability, or loss of desire, to drink

Aetiology – Relating to the cause of disease

Afferent – Carrying towards (e.g. cerebellar afferent neurones carry impulses to the cerebellum)

Agnosia – Inability to recognise objects

Agraphia – Inability to write

Akinesia – Loss, or slowness, of movement

Alexia – Inability to read

Amnesia – Loss of memory

Anastomosis – Intercommunication between vessels (e.g. circulus arteriosus or circle of Willis)

Aneurysm – Abnormal dilatation of an artery

Angioma – Congenital swollen collection of blood vessels

Angiography – Demonstration of the arterial system after injection of an opaque medium

Anomia – Inability to name objects

Antidiuretic – An agent that reduces the volume of urine produced by the kidney

Aphagia – Inability, or loss of desire, to eat

Aphasia – Loss of ability to use language

Apraxia – Loss of skilled movements despite preservation of power, sensation and coordination

Arachnoid mater – Middle of the three meningeal layers enveloping the central nervous system

Areflexia – Loss of reflexes

Arthritis – Inflammation of one or more joints

Astrocyte (astroglial cell) – A type of neuroglial cell (q.v.) that may form the blood–brain-barrier

Ataxia – Loss of ability to coordinate voluntary movements

Atrophy – Wasting or degeneration

Axon – The nerve fibre carrying impulses away from the cell body

Baroreceptor – Neuronal sensory ending that detects changes in arterial blood pressure

Biopsy – Tissue sample taken from a patient for the diagnosis of disease

Blood–brain barrier – A selectively permeable barrier between the circulating blood and the brain believed to be formed by astrocytes

Bulimia – Overeating disorder

Bradykinesia – Slowness of movement

Brain stem – The stalk-like portion of the brain connecting the cerebral hemispheres with the spinal cord

Bulbar palsy – Weakness of tongue, pharynx and larynx resulting from disease of the lower cranial nerves

Cataract – Opacity of the lens of the eye, leading to deterioration of vision

Cell body – The part of the neurone that contains the nucleus and possesses dendritic and axonal processes

Central nervous system – The brain and spinal cord

Cephalic – Relating to the head

Cerebrum – The largest, most highly developed part of the brain comprising two cerebral hemispheres

Cerebrospinal fluid (CSF) – The clear watery fluid that surrounds the brain and spinal cord

Chemoreceptor – Neuronal sensory ending that detects changes in the chemical composition of circulating blood

Chiasma – Decussation or crossing over of nerve fibres (e.g. optic chiasma)

Chorea – Involuntary, abnormal movements of the face and limbs

Collateral – A side-branch of a nerve or blood vessel

Coma – Prolonged and unnatural state of unconsciousness

Computed tomography (CT) – Imaging technique utilising X-rays to visualise the structure of the nervous system

Concussion – Loss of consciousness caused by head injury

Contralateral – Relating to the opposite side

Contusion – Bruising

Convulsion – Involuntary contraction or spasm of muscles

Cordotomy – Neurosurgical procedure to destroy specific pathways in the spinal cord

Craniopharyngioma – Congenital tumour of the base of the brain

Craniotomy – Neurosurgical procedure to open the cranial cavity

Cushing's disease – Overgrowth of the adrenal glands causing excessive release of corticosteroid hormones

Decussation – Crossing over of nerve fibres from one side of the CNS to the other (e.g. pyramidal decussation)

Dementia – Loss of mental abilities

Demyelination – Loss of the myelin sheath surrounding neuronal axons

Dendrite – Branching process of a neurone that receives information from other neurones and conducts electrical changes to the cell body

Diabetes insipidus – Failure of the posterior pituitary gland causing reduced release of antidiuretic hormone

Diabetes mellitus – A disorder of carbohydrate metabolism caused by lack of insulin

Dorsal root ganglion – Location of cell bodies of primary afferent neurones entering the spinal cord through the dorsal roots of spinal nerves

Dura mater – Outermost of the three meningeal layers that envelop the central nervous system

Dysarthria – Inability to pronounce

Dysphagia – Inability to swallow

Dysphonia – Inability to produce the voice

Echocardiography – The use of ultrasound to display the action of the heart

Efferent – Carrying away from (e.g. striatal efferent fibres carry impulses away from the striatum)

Electroencephalography (EEG) – Technique to detect the surface electrical activity of the brain

Electromyography – Technique to determine the electrical activity of muscles

Emetic – Causing nausea and vomiting

Encephalopathy – Disorder of the brain

Entrapment neuropathy – Nerve injury caused by compression of a nerve within a tunnel or at a change in direction

Ependymal cells (ependyma) – Epithelial cells lining the ventricular system

Epilepsy – Paroxysmal attack of disturbed consciousness and sensorimotor function resulting from abnormal electrophysiological discharges of the brain

Fasciculation – Spontaneous contraction of denervated motor units, visible on inspection

Fasciculus – Bundle of nerve fibres (e.g. medial longitudinal fasciculus)

Febrile – Refers to raised body temperature (fever)

Fibrillation – Spontaneous contraction of denervated muscle fibres, detected on electromyography

Foramen – An opening (e.g. foramen magnum)

Ganglion – A collection of nerve cell bodies outside the CNS (e.g. dorsal root ganglion)

General paralysis of the insane (GPI) – Disease of the frontal lobes caused by late neurosyphilis

Glia – see Neuroglia

Glioma – Tumour derived from glial cells

Haematoma – Blood clot

Haemorrhage – Escape of blood from a ruptured blood vessel

Hallucination – Abnormal perceptual experience

Hemianopia – Loss of sight affecting one half of the visual field (e.g. bitemporal hemianopia)

Hemiparesis – Weakness of one side of the body

Hemiplegia – see Hemiparesis

Hepatolenticular degeneration (Wilson's disease) – Inherited disease of copper metabolism affecting the liver and brain

Herpes zoster – Virus causing shingles (q.v.)

Huntington's disease – Inherited degenerative disease of the brain causing chorea (q.v.) and dementia (q.v.)

Hydrocephalus – Abnormal amount of cerebrospinal fluid within the ventricles of the brain

Hyperacusis – Increased hearing sensitivity

Hyperreflexia – Abnormal increase in reflex activity

Hypertonia – Abnormal increase in muscle tone

Hypertrophy – Enlargement of tissues

Hypothyroidism – Underactivity of the thyroid gland causing reduced release of thyroid hormone

Hypotonia – Abnormal decrease in muscle tone

Idiopathic – Of unknown cause

Infarction – Death of tissue resulting from impairment of its circulation

Intervertebral – Between two vertebrae

Ipsilateral – Relating to the same side

Kinaesthesia – Perception of movement

Lamina – A thin layer (e.g. internal medullary lamina)

Lesion – Site of disease or damage

Lobectomy – Surgical resection of lobe of the brain

Lumen – A space or cavity

Lymphoma – Tumour of the lymphoid system

Magnetic resonance imaging (MRI) – Technique to image structure that does not employ ionising radiation

Mastication – The act of chewing

Miosis – Pupillary constriction

Meninges – connective tissue sheaths surrounding the CNS, namely dura mater, arachnoid mater and pia mater

Meningitis – Inflammation of the meninges

Meningioma – A tumour arising from the fibrous coverings (meninges) of the brain

Metastasis – Spread of tumour to distant sites

Microglia – A type of neuroglial cell (q.v.), having a mainly phagocytic function in the response to brain damage or injury

Migraine – Paroxysmal headache

Motor neurone disease – Degenerative disease of upper and lower motor neurones, causing paralysis

Multiple sclerosis – Immune disease of the CNS, causing relapsing disorder of nervous function

Muscular dystrophy – Inherited degeneration of muscles, causing progressive paralysis

Myasthenia gravis – Immune disorder of the neuromuscular junction, causing muscular fatigue

Myelin – A sheath of protein and phospholipid around the axons of certain neurones

Myopathy – Disease of muscle

Narcolepsy – Paroxysmal sleep attacks

Necrosis – Death of tissue

Neoplasia – Tumorous overgrowth of tissue

Neurofibromatosis – Inherited disease causing tumours of meninges, CNS, peripheral nerves and skin

Neuroglia (neuroglial cell) – non-neural supporting cells of the CNS comprised of oligodendrocytes, astrocytes, microglia and ependymal cells (q.v.)

Neuroma – Tumour derived from nerve cells

Neurone – The principle functional cell of the nervous system, specialised to integrate and transmit nerve impulses

Neuropathy – Disease of nerve cells

Neurosyphilis – Infection of the nervous system by a spirochaete

Neurotransmitter – Chemical substance stored within vesicles (q.v.) in presynaptic nerve endings and released on depolarisation to act upon postsynaptic receptors

Nociception – Sensitivity to noxious stimuli

Nucleus – Structure within a cell that contains chromosomal DNA; also a collection of nerve cell bodies within the CNS (e.g. dentate nucleus)

Nystagmus – To-and-fro movements of the eyes

Oedema – Swelling caused by accumulated fluid

Oligodendrocyte (oligodendroglia) – A type of neuroglial cell (q.v.) that produces the myelin sheath in the CNS

Oligodendroglioma – Tumour derived from oligodendroglia

Ophthalmoscopy – Clinical examination of the eye with an ophthalmoscope

Pallidum – Globus pallidus

Palsy – Weakness

Papilloedema – Swelling of the optic nerve(s)

Paraesthesia – Tingling sensations ('pins and needles')

Paralysis – Muscle weakness of varying severity

Paraphasia – Use of incorrect word

Paraplegia – Weakness or paralysis of the legs

Paresis – Muscular weakness

Parkinson's disease – Disease of the basal ganglia causing akinesia (q.v.), rigidity (q.v.) and tremor (q.v.)

Paroxysm – Sudden attack

Peripheral nervous system – All parts of the nervous system excluding the brain and spinal cord (CNS)

Photophobia – Intolerance to light

Pia mater – Innermost of the three meningeal layers that envelop the central nervous system

Plexus – Structure consisting of interwoven nerves (e.g. brachial plexus) or blood vessels (e.g. choroid plexus)

Poliomyelitis – Viral infection of motor neurones of the spinal cord and brain stem

Positron emission tomography (PET) – Technique for imaging the function of the brain

Prolapse – Displacement from normal anatomical position

Proprioception – The detection of position and movement of body parts

Pseudobulbar palsy – Weakness of the tongue, pharynx and larynx caused by disease of the corticobulbar tracts

Psychosis – Abnormal mental state with altered precepts (hallucinations) and false ideas (delusions)

Ptosis – Abnormal drooping of the eyelid

Quadriplegia – Paralysis affecting all four limbs

Radiculopathy – Disease of the nerve roots

Receptor – Specialised element of the cell membrane that binds neurotransmitter substances (or exogenous drugs) bringing about a change in membrane permeability or an intracellular response

Resting potential – The electrical potential across the membrane of a nerve cell at rest

Rheumatic fever – Immune disease of the joints, heart and brain following bacterial infection

Rigidity – Increased resistance to passive movement of the limbs throughout their range

Schizophrenia – Disease of the brain causing psychosis (q.v.)

Seizure – Sudden disturbance of consciousness or sensorimotor function

Shingles – Infection of the ganglia of cranial and spinal nerves by herpes zoster virus (q.v.)

Single photon emission tomography (SPECT) – Technique for imaging the function of the brain

Somatic – Relating to body parts other than the viscera

Somatotopic – The orderly representation of body parts in the CNS

Spasticity – Increased resistance to passive movement of the limbs when muscles are initially stretched

Spondylosis – Degeneration of the spine

Stroke – Sudden neurological deficit caused by disease of the circulation to the brain

Sydenham's chorea – Manifestation of rheumatic fever (q.v.) affecting the basal ganglia and causing involuntary movements

Synapse – The gap between neurones across which nerve impulses pass by release of a neurotransmitter

Synaptic vesicle – Structure within the presynaptic ending that contains neurotransmitter substance which is released on depolarisation

Syncope – Fainting attack

Syndrome – Group of signs and symptoms which characterise a disease

Syringobulbia – Expanding cavity (syrinx) within the medulla

Syringomyelia – Expanding cavity within the spinal cord

Syrinx – An abnormal cavity in the spinal cord

Thalamotomy – Neurosurgical destruction of part of the thalamus

Terminal bouton – specialised presynaptic ending of an axon

Thrombosis – Coagulation of blood in artery or vein

Tract – An aggregation of nerve cell processes having more or less the same origin and destination (e.g. corticospinal tract)

Tremor – Trembling of head or limbs

Tumour – A swelling or morbid enlargement; a mass of abnormal tissue resulting from uncontrolled cell growth (neoplasm)

Vesicle – see Synaptic vesicle

Index